Lois S. Esparza

THE UNFAMILIAR MENOPAUSE

What every woman should know

Empowering Women's Health Through Science-supported technique, Support, and Self-Advancement

TABLE OF CONTENT

ABOUT THE CREATOR

Lois s. Esparza,A notable figure of the nineties Brit Pop scene, Lois s. Esparza is a previous music industry PR, occasion organizer, and creator turned business person, creator, and backer for menopause.

Brought into the world in Guernsey, UK on fourteenth Walk 1966, to developer, Samuel Esparza and secretary, Christiana Esparza, Lois emigrated to South Africa at nine years old. She got back to the UK three years after the fact, going to Oxford Sibford Tuition-based school until she was fifteen, preceding moving to London.

Her initial yearning was to be a veterinary medical caretaker, and she accomplished the necessary capabilities to move into this profession. But, Lois' initial life and vocation were molded by the London music scene, tracking down her direction into music the executives, coming full circle in her work at Creation Records.

In 1997, she wedded performer, Thaddeus Imprint, bringing forth their little girl, Gabrielle Imprint at Portland Clinic in 2000.

From the music business, Lois proceeded to work effectively as an originator, having planned the two scarves and backdrop for the extravagance retail chain, Freedom London. Her most memorable inside plan client was Victoria Beckham, and her adoration for both style and inside plan proceeds right up to the present day.

Be that as it may, Lois' actual work seemingly started in 2016. In the wake of turning 50, she started to encounter menopausal side effects and was stunned at the absence of help made accessible for ladies right now in their lives. From here, she made it her main goal to change perspectives, break marks of shame and assist ladies with feeling enabled around everything menopause.

Following the fruitful send-off of Lois' Menopause, a space devoted to straight-to-the-point and open conversations around the subject, in 2018, Lois sent off a scope of menopause items, zeroed in on private consideration, skin health management, and nourishment.

She proceeds with her work as a representative regarding the matter, showing up on worldwide Programs and driving discussions at associations, for example, Unfamiliar and Republic Office, BBC, and John Lewis and Accomplices.

Having involved her menopause as an opportunity to rethink and reset, Lois' message encompassing it is one of reexamination. Empowering ladies to embrace this new part of their lives, she wants to instruct and rouse, while breaking restrictions fully backed by clinical experts, and deal tips to assist ladies with assuming command over their lives.

Lois is likewise a web-based reporter for Red magazine and was named by the distribution as one of their main

20 Profession Shifters in 2017. In 2018, she was given the Rousing Well-known Person of the Year grant by the Motivational Authority Trust.

Close by her work on the menopause, Lois s. Esparza is energetic about creatures. From saving a canine in the city of Camden in 1997 to turning into a diplomat for Little Guy Help, Lois keeps on utilizing her foundation to stand up as a functioning campaigner for basic entitlements and supports various creature noble causes. In 2004, she campaigned for Hostile to Fox Hunting, and in 2020 assumed a key part in getting Lucy's Regulation passed, prohibiting all outsider doggy deals in Britain.

Her indispensable work on both menopause and basic entitlements proceeds.

DISCLAIMER

DESCRIPTION

Filling a vast opening in menopause care, all that a lady has to be aware of to flourish during her hormonal change and then some, as well as the devices to assist her with charging her well-being at this urgent life stage — by the smash hit creator of The Galveston Diet. Menopause is inescapable, however it isn't to endure it! This is the engaging way to deal with self-backing that spearheading ladies' wellbeing advocate Lois s. Esparza takes for ladies amidst hormonal change in The Unfamiliar Menopause. An exhaustive, legitimate book of science-upheld data and lived insight, it covers each lady's necessities:

From changes in your appearance and rest examples to neurological, outer muscle, mental, and sexual issues, an extensive start-to-finish tool stash of science-supported choices for adapting to side effects.

How to intervene against the dangers related to your body's regular drop in estrogen creation, including diabetes, dementia, Alzheimer's, osteoporosis, cardiovascular illness, and weight gain.

Step-by-step instructions to advocate and plan for yearly midlife health visits, including inquiries for your PCP and how to demand entire life care.

The extremely most recent examination on the advantages and symptoms of chemical substitution treatment.

Outfitting ladies with the ability to get energetic well-being and prosperity until the end of their lives, The Unfamiliar Menopause makes certain to turn into the guidebook for midlife health for the current and people tomorrow.

The significance of grasping menopause

It is basic to see menopause as only one point in a continuum of life stages. A lady's well-being status entering the perimenopausal period will to a great not be entirely settled by earlier well-being and conceptive history, way of life, and ecological elements. Perimenopausal and postmenopausal side effects can be troublesome to individual and expert lives, and changes related to menopause will influence a lady's well-being as she ages. In this way, perimenopausal care assumes a significant part in the advancement of sound maturing and personal satisfaction.

Menopause can be a significant change according to a social viewpoint, as well as a natural one. Socially, a lady's insight into menopause might be impacted by orientation standards, and familial and sociocultural elements, including how female maturing and the menopausal progress are seen in her way of life.

The worldwide populace of postmenopausal ladies is developing. In 2021, ladies matured 50 and more than represented 26% of all ladies and young ladies universally. This was high from 22% 10 years previously. Additionally, ladies are living longer.

Universally, a lady who matured 60 years in 2019 could hope to live on normally for an additional 21 years. Menopause can offer a significant chance to reevaluate one's well-being, way of life, and objectives.

General wellbeing challenges connected with menopause

Perimenopausal ladies need admittance to quality well-being administrations and networks and frameworks that can uphold them. Sadly, both mindfulness and admittance to menopause-related data and administrations remain a huge test in many nations. Menopause is frequently not examined inside families, networks, working environments, or medical services settings.

Ladies may not realize that side effects they experience are connected with menopause, or that there are directing and treatment choices that can assist with reducing uneasiness. Those encountering menopausal side effects might feel humiliated or embarrassed to notice their encounters and request support.

Medical services suppliers may not be prepared to perceive perimenopausal and post-menopausal side effects and advise patients on therapy choices and remaining sound after the menopausal change. Menopause right now gets restricted consideration in the preparation of educational plans for some medical services laborers.

The sexual prosperity of menopausal ladies is neglected in numerous nations. This implies that normal gynecological impacts of menopause, including vaginal dryness and torment during intercourse, may go neglected. Likewise, more seasoned ladies may not view themselves as in danger of physically communicated contaminations, including HIV[iii], or may not be guided by their suppliers to rehearse more secure sex or get tried.

Numerous states don't have well-being policies and funding for the incorporation of menopause-related analysis, guiding, and treatment administrations as a feature of their regularly accessible administrations. Menopause-related administrations are a specific test in settings where there are frequently other dire and contending needs for well-being subsidizing.

INTRODUCTION

Menopause is a characteristic organic interaction that denotes the finish of a lady's regenerative years. It normally happens in ladies in their late 40s or mid-50s, however can likewise happen prior or later. Menopause is described by a diminishing in the development of estrogen and progesterone, which are the chemicals liable for directing the period.

The side effects of menopause can change from one lady to another, however, a few normal side effects incorporate hot blazes, night sweats, state of mind swings, vaginal dryness, and trouble resting. These side effects can be awkward and problematic to day-to-day existence, driving numerous ladies to look for treatment to ease them.

One part of menopause that is frequently neglected is the personal and mental effect it can have on ladies. The progress to menopause can be a difficult time for some ladies, as they might encounter sensations of misfortune, bitterness, and nervousness about maturing and the progressions occurring in their bodies. This close-to-home part of menopause is frequently alluded to as the "new menopause," as it is a time of vulnerability and change for some ladies.

In a pugnacious paper, it tends to be contended that the profound and mental parts of menopause are similarly pretty much as significant as the actual side effects, and ought to be focused on more consideration in conversations about menopause. While there is an abundance of data accessible about the actual side effects of menopause and treatment choices, there is less spotlight on the profound and mental effect of this change.

Research has shown that ladies going through menopause are at an expanded gamble of creating sadness and uneasiness, as well as encountering changes in their confidence and self-perception. These close-to-home and mental changes can essentially affect a lady's personal satisfaction and general prosperity.

Medical services suppliers and society all in all really must perceive and address the profound and mental parts of menopause, notwithstanding the actual side effects. Ladies going through menopause ought to be upheld and urged to look for help assuming that they are battling inwardly, and ought to be furnished with assets and data to assist them with exploring this difficult time. All in all, the "new menopause" alludes to the profound mental effect of menopause on ladies, which is much of the time disregarded in conversations about this normal progress. By recognizing and tending to the close-to-home parts of menopause, we can more readily uphold ladies going through this progress and assist them with exploring this time of progress with effortlessness and flexibility.

MY NEW MENOPAUSE LIFE

Menopause is a characteristic stage in a lady's life that denotes the finish of her regenerative years. It is a period of huge physical and profound changes, as the body acclimates to diminishing degrees of estrogen and progesterone. I as of late entered this new period of life, and it has been an excursion of self-disclosure and variation.

As I explored through the beginning phases of menopause, I encountered a scope of side effects that were both testing and new. Hot glimmers, night sweats, state of mind swings, and weariness turned into an ordinary piece of my day-to-day existence. These side effects frequently left me feeling disappointed and overpowered, as I battled to adapt to the progressions occurring in my body.

Despite the difficulties, I realized that I expected to assume command over my well-being and prosperity during this momentary period. I started to teach myself about menopause and its consequences for the body, searching out data from trustworthy sources and medical care experts. Outfitted with information, I had the option to arrive at informed conclusions about my well-being and way of life decisions.

One of the main parts of dealing with my menopause side effects was taking on a solid way of life. I zeroed in on eating a reasonable eating routine, practicing consistently, and getting sufficient rest and unwinding. These straightforward changes assisted me with feeling more stimulated and adjusted, and I saw a huge improvement in my general prosperity.

Notwithstanding the way of life transforms, I additionally investigated elective treatments and medicines to assist with mitigating my menopause side effects. Needle therapy, homegrown enhancements, and care rehearsal all assumed a part in supporting my physical and profound well-being during this season of change. These all-encompassing methodologies assisted me with feeling more on top of my body and brain and gave me a feeling of strengthening and command over my menopause experience.

As I keep on exploring my new menopause life, I'm appreciative of the chance to gain and develop from this extraordinary experience. Menopause has helped me to embrace change, pay attention to my body, and focus on taking care of myself. It has likewise helped me to remember the flexibility and strength that exists in me, as I face the difficulties and vulnerabilities of this new period of life.

My menopause process has been a period of self-disclosure and variation. By assuming command over my well-being and prosperity, taking on a sound way of life, and investigating elective treatments, I have had the option to explore this momentary period with effortlessness and flexibility. Menopause might be a difficult time, yet it is likewise a period of development, strengthening, and change. I'm thankful for the examples and encounters that menopause has brought into my life, and I anticipate embracing the following section with certainty and good faith.

Menopause is a characteristic organic cycle that denotes the finish of a lady's conceptive years. It regularly happens in ladies between the ages of 45 and 55, although it can happen before or later for certain ladies. Menopause is portrayed by a lessening in the development of estrogen and progesterone, which are the chemicals liable for managing the monthly cycle.

As a lady moving toward menopause, I ended up confronting various physical and personal difficulties. I encountered hot glimmers, night sweats, state of mind swings, and trouble resting. I additionally saw changes in my skin, hair, and weight. These side effects caused me to feel awkward and hesitant, and I battled to adapt to the progressions occurring in my body.

To explore this temporary period in my life, I realized that I expected to assume command over my well-being and prosperity. I started exploring menopause and its consequences for the body, searching out data from legitimate sources like clinical diaries and medical care experts. I found out about the significance of keeping a sound eating regimen, practicing routinely, and overseeing pressure to reduce a portion of the side effects related to menopause.

I additionally searched for help from different ladies who were going through menopause or had previously gone through it. I joined web-based discussions and care groups where I could share my encounters and gain from other people who were confronting comparable difficulties. Associating with different ladies who comprehended what I was going through assisted me with feeling not so much alone but rather more engaged in assuming responsibility for my well-being.

As well as searching out data and backing, I likewise tried to focus on taking care of myself during this time. I made a point to get customary check-ups with my medical services supplier, and I examined my side effects and concerns transparently with them. I likewise set aside a few minutes for exercises that gave me pleasure and unwinding, like yoga, contemplation, and investing energy with friends and family.

Through my proactive way of dealing with self-headway during menopause, I had the option to more readily deal with my side effects and further develop my general prosperity.

In conclusion, menopause is a characteristic and unavoidable piece of a lady's life, yet it doesn't need to be a period of misery or decline. By adopting a proactive strategy for self-progression during menopause, ladies can enable themselves to assume command over their well-being and prosperity. Through training, backing, and taking care of oneself, ladies can explore this temporary period with certainty and effortlessness.

WHO REACTION

WHO thinks that social, mental, and actual well-being support during the menopausal change and after menopause ought to be a vital piece of medical care. WHO is focused on expanding comprehension of menopause by:

bringing issues to light of menopause and its effect on ladies at individual and cultural levels, as well as on nations' well-being and financial turn of events; upholding the incorporation of conclusion, treatment, and advice connected with the board of menopausal side effects as a component of general well-being inclusion; advancing the consideration of preparing on menopause and treatment choices in pre-administration educational programs for well-being laborers; and underlining a day-to-day existence course way to deal with well-being and prosperity (counting sexual well-being and prosperity), by guaranteeing that ladies approach fitting well-being data and administrations to advance solid maturing and an excellent life previously, during, and after menopause.
Notes:

1) While most individual encounters with menopause connect with cisgender ladies (who were conceived female and recognized as female), transsexual men and certain individuals who are distinguished as neither men nor ladies additionally experience menopause.

This reality sheet alludes to "ladies" in arrangement with the accessible information, which doesn't regularly distinguish orientation character. There is a lack of promptly accessible information on trans and orientation different encounters of menopause. Trans and orientation different individuals have remarkable age-related well-being need that clinicians ought to consider, including reference to expert administrations when important.

2) Although menopause isn't an illness, this reality sheet alludes to the perimenopausal and postmenopausal encounters of ladies as side effects since they can bring about a degree of uneasiness that influences their satisfaction.

Key realities
Menopause is one point in a continuum of life stages for ladies and imprints the finish of their regenerative years. After menopause, a lady can't become pregnant, except in uncommon situations when particular rich medicines are utilized.
Most ladies experience menopause between the ages of 45 and 55 years as a characteristic piece of organic maturing.
Menopause is brought about by the deficiency of ovarian follicular capability and a decrease in flowing blood estrogen levels.
The menopausal progress can be slow, normally starting with changes in the period. 'Perimenopause' alludes to the period from when these signs are first noticed and close one year after the last feminine period.

Perimenopause can most recent quite a long while and can influence physical, profound, mental, and social prosperity.
Different non-hormonal and hormonal medications can help lighten perimenopausal side effects.
Menopause can be an outcome of careful operations.
How menopause happens
For most ladies, menopause is set apart toward the finish of month to month feminine cycle (otherwise called a feminine period or 'period') because of loss of ovarian follicular capability. This implies that the ovaries quit delivering eggs for preparation.

The routineness and length of the period differ across a lady's regenerative life expectancy, however, the age at which normal menopause happens is by and large somewhere in the range of 45 and 55 years for ladies around the world.

Regular menopause is considered to have happened following 12 continuous months without a period for which there could be no other clear physiological or neurotic reason and without a trace of clinical mediation.

A few ladies experience menopause prior (before 40 years old). This 'untimely menopause' might be a direct result of specific chromosomal irregularities, immune system issues, or other obscure causes.

It is preposterous to expect to foresee when a singular lady will encounter menopause, although there are relationship between the age at menopause and certain segments, well-being, and hereditary elements.

Menopause can likewise be initiated as a result of surgeries that include expulsion of the two ovaries or clinical mediations that cause the end of ovarian capability (for instance radiation treatment or chemotherapy).

Numerous ladies have proactively quit discharging before menopause, for instance, the people who have had specific surgeries (hysterectomy or careful expulsion of their uterine coating) as well as those utilizing specific hormonal contraceptives and different meds that cause rare or missing periods. They might in any case encounter different changes connected with the menopausal progress.

Changes related to menopause
The hormonal changes related to menopause can influence physical, profound, mental, and social prosperity. The side effects experienced during and following the menopausal progress shift considerably from one individual to another. Some have scarcely any side effects. For other people, side effects can be extreme and influence everyday exercise and personal satisfaction. Some can encounter side effects for quite a long time.

Side effects related to menopause include:

hot flushes and night sweats. Hot flushes allude to an unexpected sensation of intensity in the face, neck, and chest, frequently joined by flushing of the skin, sweat (perspiring), palpitations, and intense sensations of actual distress which can most recent a few minutes; changes in the routineness and stream of the feminine cycle, coming full circle in discontinuance of period; vaginal dryness, torment during sex, and incontinence; trouble resting/a sleeping disorder; and

changes in state of mind, despondency, and additionally uneasiness.

Body synthesis and cardiovascular gambling can likewise be impacted. Ladies' benefit over men as far as cardiovascular illness bit by bit vanishes with the huge decrease in estrogen levels after menopause. Menopause can likewise bring about the debilitating of the pelvic help structures, expanding the gamble of pelvic organ prolapse. Deficiency of bone thickness at menopause is a huge supporter of higher paces of osteoporosis and cracks.

There are various non-hormonal and hormonal medications that can assist with the lightening side effects of menopause. Side effects that affect well-being and prosperity ought to be examined with a medical care supplier to distinguish accessible administration choices, with the thought of clinical history, values, and inclinations.

Pregnancy is as yet conceivable during perimenopause. Contraception is prescribed to keep away from accidental pregnancy until the following 12 sequential months without a feminine cycle. Pregnancy after menopause is impossible without richness treatment that includes the utilization of benefactor eggs or recently frozen incipient organisms.

During perimenopause and following menopause, it is as yet conceivable to secure physically sent diseases (STIs), including HIV, through unprotected sexual contact, including oral, butt-centric, and vaginal sex. The diminishing of the vaginal wall after menopause builds the possibility of injuries and tears, subsequently expanding the gamble of HIV transmission during vaginal sex.

Menopause is a characteristic organic interaction that denotes the finish of a lady's regenerative years. It normally happens in ladies between the ages of 45 and 55, even though it can happen before or later for certain ladies. Menopause is described by a decline in the creation of estrogen and progesterone chemicals, which prompts the end of the feminine cycle and the finish of ripeness.

The change to menopause, known as perimenopause, can keep going for a long time and is set apart by various side effects. These side effects can incorporate hot glimmers, night sweats, mindset swings, vaginal dryness, and changes in drive.

While certain ladies might encounter just gentle side effects, others might have more extreme side effects that can altogether influence their satisfaction.

One of the most widely recognized side effects of menopause is hot glimmers, which are abrupt sensations of warmth that can cause perspiring and flushing of the skin. Hot blazes can happen whenever of day or night and can keep going for a couple of moments to a few minutes. They are believed to be brought about by changes in chemical levels that influence the internal heat level's guidelines.

One more typical side effect of menopause is vaginal dryness, which can prompt distress during sex. This is because of a reduction in estrogen levels, which can make the vaginal tissues more slender and less versatile. Ladies encountering vaginal dryness may likewise be more inclined to urinary lot diseases and other vaginal issues.

Mind-set swings are likewise a typical side effect of menopause, as fluctuating chemical levels can influence synapses in the cerebrum that manage temperament. Ladies might encounter sensations of touchiness, uneasiness, or misery during this time. It is significant for ladies encountering extreme emotional episodes to look for help from medical care suppliers or psychological wellness experts.

While menopause is a characteristic piece of the maturing system, it can in any case be a difficult time for some ladies. Ladies genuinely must deal with themselves during this process by eating a sound eating routine, practicing consistently, and getting sufficient rest. A few ladies may likewise profit from chemical substitution treatment or different medicines to assist with dealing with their side effects.

Menopause is a typical cycle that all ladies will insight as they age. While it extremely well may be a tough, with side effects like hot glimmers, vaginal dryness, and emotional episodes, there are ways of dealing with these side effects and keeping decent personal satisfaction. By looking for help from medical services suppliers and settling on a solid way of life decisions, ladies can explore the progress to menopause with effortlessness and strength.

Menopause-related drops in capability might be the consequence of regular maturing of the endocrine hub or brought about by the evacuation of the ovaries or clinical treatment that forestalls ovarian endocrine capability.

Nonetheless, menopause is likewise a neurological change, as shown by numerous trademark side effects of menopause, particularly carelessness, rest unsettling influences, modified temperament, and hot glimmers. Ovarian and cerebrum well-being are hence inseparably connected in ladies.

As estrogen levels fall, changes happen in the morphology, number, and communications between nerve cells, their glucose digestion, and quality articulation. In female creature models, low estrogen has been connected to the collection of the unusual protein amyloid-beta (Aβ), which is famous for framing plaques inside cerebrum tissue, in individuals with Alzheimer's sickness (Promotion), however likewise once in a while in ordinary individuals.

Cerebrum endocrine hub
Contingent upon the phase of menopause (pre-menopause, peri-menopause, and post-menopause), the cerebrum structure and brain network, as well as energy digestion, go through stamped changes. The cerebrum regions engaged with higher mental capabilities were generally impacted at all ages. This impact was noticed autonomous of other cardiovascular or dementia risk factors like ApoE-4 levels, hysterectomy, or the utilization of chemical substitution.

In post-menopausal ladies, the earliest change in the mind has all the earmarks of being a fall in how much glucose is utilized by the cerebrum, showing diminished cerebrum action. This is because of falling estrogen levels, this chemical being essential for mind glucose digestion.

Neuroscientist Lisa Mosconi, the creator of a concentrate on this part of menopause, makes sense of: "When estrogen doesn't initiate the nerve center accurately, the mind can't manage internal heat level accurately. So those hot glimmers that ladies get - that is the nerve center. Then, at that point, there's the brainstem accountable for rest and wake. At the point when estrogen doesn't enact the brainstem accurately, we experience difficulty resting. On the other hand, it's the amygdala, the profound focus of the mind near the hippocampus, the memory focus of the cerebrum. At the point when estrogen's levels ebb in these locales, we begin getting emotional episodes maybe and fail to remember things."

Dim matter volume in the mind declines also. These boundaries answer chemical substitution, in any case, recommending that the connection between the focal sensory system and endocrine hub stays dynamic for quite a while after the menopausal progress starts.

These markers of mental degradation standardized after menopause, and the dark matter volume likewise recuperated to pattern in the cerebrum regions generally worried about menopausal endocrine maturing.

Vasomotor side effects and mental debilitation

Mental degradation is normal during the progress into menopause, including side effects, for example, absent-mindedness and postponed verbal memory, decreased verbal handling speed, and debilitated verbal learning. Prior research shows that memory-related grumblings are anticipated by age, hot blazes, sorrow, sensations of stress, and the apparent degree of well-being.

Solid ladies showed slight however predictable changes in verbal memory and learning, as well as handling speed. Reassuringly, execution gets back to ordinary postmenopausally.

Vasomotor side effects (VMS) are the side effects normal for the menopausal progress however may happen previously, during, or after menopause. These side effects incorporate hot blazes and night sweats. Like mental side effects, their event doesn't reflect the falling degrees of estradiol.

As of now, it is believed that the hippocampus, parahippocampus, and different districts of the prefrontal cortex of the mind are associated with the beginning of mental degradation related to serious VMS.

VMS is related to hypertension, high blood lipid levels, an inclination towards insulin obstruction and diabetes risk, and at times a procoagulant profile. The gamble of future stroke is likewise proposed to be higher in ladies with more serious objective VMS.

VMS is additionally connected with expanded cortisol levels, at around 20 minutes following the occasion, which is known to be connected to memory impedance. These occasions may likewise frequently cause a 5% lessening in the bloodstream. Subsequently, VMS might be a determinants of cognizance at this midlife progress point.

VMS could subsequently be a gamble factor for cardiovascular sickness and mental weakness during this change, as well as the critical middle person between them.

RECUPERATION AFTER MENOPAUSE

Contrasted with guys of similar age, ladies going through menopausal progress have critical modifications in cerebrum biomarkers. The neurological changes happening close to this time cause side effects that thus trigger discouragement and nervousness, as well as Promotion, in a small part of ladies.

The progressive beginning of endocrine maturing with unconstrained menopause might permit the mind to conform to and make up for the deficiency of estrogen and estrogen receptor movement. This resetting of the mind might make sense of why side effects like hot flashes ease 2-7 years from their beginning.

Neuroimaging affirms these discoveries. In the post-menopausal lady, dim matter volume gets back to business as usual, particularly in regions worried about certain sorts of memory and mental handling. As a matter of fact, in postmenopausal ladies, the dim matter volume was like that of guys of similar age and expanded throughout the following two years.

This volume is additionally related to rising memory scores in a space called the precuneus which shows underlying changes during the menopausal progress. This is controlled by estrogen, and changes during pregnancy, one more one-of-a-kind female stage related with neurologic and endocrine changes.

White matter volume falls during menopause and doesn't recuperate from there on. Notwithstanding, contrasted with guys, ladies going through or past menopause showed higher primary availability and myelination, which might demonstrate that the brain networks in these districts are more productive following the beginning of menopause.

Energy digestion
Estrogen is critical to glucose usage in the mind. During the menopausal progress, the digestion of glucose in the cerebrum originally dropped however at that point steadied at another level, again recommending versatile changes. ATP levels rose after menopause, as did worldwide proportions of discernment. Mitochondrial recuperation might make sense of how ladies can go on with flawless mental capacities after menopause.

Chemical treatment and insight
Does chemical treatment assist with saving discernment? Dr. Mosconi says that chemicals might assist with further developing insight. In late postmenopausal ladies, the gamble of dementia is higher with consolidated estrogen-progesterone treatment, yet unaltered when estrogen alone is utilized. In early post-menopause, in any case, chemicals showed no consequences for perception.
She sums up, "By and large, HT's viability is remembered to rely upon the timing of treatment commencement as for age at menopause, with benefits

relating to early inception, particularly after instigated menopause."

Chemicals might collaborate with high body weight to create the contrary result. Alternately, the way of life and wellness might connect decidedly with estrogen, particularly in the long haul. Some examination proposes that nearby estrogen union inside the cerebrum happens autonomously of estrogen available for use after menopause, keeping up with hippocampal capability.
Menopause itself, in this way, doesn't proclaim a drop in mental capacity, in contrast to the temporary time frame itself. Ladies improve at mental errands than men over their grown-up life, including during dementia! All things being equal, menopause might be thought of as "a powerful neurological progress that reshapes the brain scene of the female cerebrum during midlife endocrine maturing, [with] a versatile cycle serving the change into late life."

Further perusing will be important to comprehend what hereditary elements and ailments mean for mental capability during menopause. When Lisa Mosconi began concentrating on the effect of menopause on the mind, she understood two significant realities.
To begin with, not many cerebrum studies checked out menopause by any means. Second, the not many that did took a gander at more seasoned ladies who were far beyond menopause.

"Menopause had been for the most part concentrated on with regards to its impact on the mind sometime later," says Mosconi, the overseer of the Weill Cornell ladies' cerebrum drive and writer of the approaching book The Menopause Cerebrum. "More like an product than a process."Mosconi is important for a river of expertise studying the menopause-cerebrum association. While there's something else to learn, obviously menopause should be reevaluated as a regenerative wellbeing occasion as well as a neurological one. Historically, this association has been underrated. Many variables have postponed our comprehension, yet to summarize it: "Ageism and sexism and their convergence likely added to this not being important," says Pauline Maki, a teacher, and head of the ladies' psychological wellness research program, at the College of Illinois at Chicago.

She has seen a flood of interest of late, extending from the clinical foundation to the big-name domain, in completely figuring out menopause and normalizing it.

"I've been in this field for the greater part of my life, and it surprises me what an ocean change there is at present," Maki says.
Ladies are requesting to find out about what's in store, and suppliers need further developed direction for their patients. This mirrors a bleak standard: research proposes that 60% to 86% of ladies look for clinical consideration for their menopause side effects, however, many feel misjudged and disheartened after their arrangements. Most ladies under 40 are

underinformed about menopause, and just a little cut of suppliers feel ready to sufficiently respond to their inquiries.

An expanded comprehension of the cerebrum menopause association can assist individuals with exploring this period in a manner that advances mind well-being and prosperity. This is the very thing that we know up to this point - and why there's more work to be finished.

What befalls the cerebrum during menopause Menopause comprises three phases: perimenopause, the long-term change paving the way to an individual's last period; menopause; and postmenopause, or every one of the years past menopause. It's a characteristic piece of maturing and denotes the finish of having the option to bear youngsters. During this cycle, ovaries quit delivering eggs and the creation of estrogen and progesterone chemicals declines.
The menopause stage is affirmed when an individual has missed their period for a very long time, however, side effects can happen all through. Around 70% of ladies experience neurological side effects during the menopausal progress, says Emily Jacobs, an academic partner at the College of California at St Nick Barbara and overseer of the Ann S Arbors ladies' mind wellbeing drive. While generally menopause was related exclusively to the ovaries, it's currently perceived that side effects, for example, hot blazes, distraction, state of

mind changes, and a sleeping disorder are neurological side effects.
The mind goes through this progress "since it's a good idea to do as such", says Mosconi. The neurons that help ovulation and empower pregnancy are not generally required. It's the cerebrum's opportunity to recalibrate, which can prompt some distress yet in addition some advantages."The decrease in hormonal changes can prompt a more steady temperament and close-to-home prosperity for certain," Mosconi says.

In 2017, Mosconi and her partners distributed the primary mind imaging study exhibiting a distinction in cerebrum movement between premenopausal ladies and people who are at the perimenopausal and postmenopausal stages. Her 2021 review, the biggest assessment of the menopausal mind to date, further showed significant contrasts in cerebrum structure, how various pieces of the mind speak with one another, and energy digestion across the menopause stages. Fundamentally, large numbers of these progressions are impermanent - like a dunk in dark matter volume in the precuneus, a piece of the cerebrum engaged with memory - and the mind attempts to make up for these progressions through expanded bloodstream and energy creation.

This examination shows that these progressions happen given menopause, not simply maturing, and points out the way that while menopause is a regenerative change express, it's likewise a neurological progress.

WHAT MENOPAUSE CAN MEAN FOR MEMORY?

During menopause, certain individuals report encountering mind haze - mental blips described by distraction. All things considered, during menopause, says Maki. How widespread this experience and the factors that lead to it are as yet discussed, she makes sense of. (Since ladies regularly beat men with regards to memory, "they're simply declining to the degree of men", makes sense to Jacobs.)

Plunging chemical levels might make sense of why memory issues occur for some. Be that as it may, shockingly, hot blazes might be a preferred pointer over estrogen levels of those who will have these mental issues. "What we find is that the more hot blazes ladies have, the more awful their memory," says Maki. Maki is looking at why this affiliation exists, yet one chance is the ongoing lack of sleep that can go with hot glimmers; great rest is basic for a solid mind. Early exploration recommends memory execution returns when hot glimmers are dealt with.

In 2023, in the wake of examining the blood of study members, Maki and her group likewise tracked down a relationship between continuous hot glimmers and an improved probability of having Alzheimer's sickness biomarkers. She's fast to alert that this doesn't imply that an individual will foster Alzheimer's assuming that they have hot glimmers or feel careless during menopause. However, the connection merits analysis because postmenopausal ladies address 70% of individuals with Alzheimer's sickness.

The mental neuroscientist Rachel Buckley, an associate teacher at Harvard Clinical School, investigates likely connections among menopause and Alzheimer's infection. The primary indications of the mind issue can show up at about similar time ladies start menopause, proposing the hormonal occasion could have suggestions for sickness risk. A recent report distributed by Buckley and her group recommends that two variables are connected with a more noteworthy probability of having raised degrees of tau, a protein that is a biomarker of Alzheimer's sickness: early menopause, and a long defer between the beginning of menopause and the beginning of chemical treatment, a menopause therapy.

"Neither of those things implies you explicitly will get dementia," Buckley stresses.

This data can, nonetheless, lead to a superior comprehension of who is bound to foster Alzheimer's illness and, for the time being, further develop the way that specialists screen their patients, makes sense of. It likewise highlights how significant it is for individuals to know about and impart their side effects and have a way of life that supports mind well-being.

INSTRUCTIONS TO DEAL WITH THE MENOPAUSE CEREBRUM

Many individuals who arrive at menopause feel they ought to "buck up and continue ahead with it", says Buckley. In any case, disregarding or making light of distress denies reality and holds ladies back from embracing medications that can help, she adds. These incorporate way-of-life changes that can begin before menopause. Keeping the cerebrum sound through diet, workout, positive social collaborations, and stress the board can set it up for future difficulties. Weighty smoking, for instance, can set off early menopause.

There are clinical choices that diminish menopausal side effects. Chemical treatment is an umbrella word for different meds that supplant estrogen, progestin, or a blend. In a 2023 explanation, the North American Menopause Society depicted chemical treatment as "the best treatment" for vasomotor side effects like hot blazes and night sweats. It's not the most ideal decision for everybody, so it merits examining this choice with a consideration supplier.

Mental conduct treatment, SSRIs, and hot glimmer drugs can ease menopause side effects as well. A great many people who experience hot blazes, says Maki, could profit from talking with their PCP about how to treat them.

What researchers need to be aware Cerebrum-related side effects, similar to memory slips, normally work after some time. In any case, how the cerebrum changes and quickly returns after menopause isn't perceived. Most investigations are review or think about ladies at various menopause stages, says Jacobs. All the more long haul concentrates on that follow a different, huge gathering of ladies from menopause til' the very end could assist researchers with estimating changes connected with explicit people after some time, she makes sense of. She is presently fostering an exhaustive menopause project with different researchers, wanting to do precisely that.
Further examination could bring about greater treatment choices, a superior comprehension of what makes a mind stronger or defenseless during menopause, and further developed direction about what's in store.
"Assuming that we comprehend what's regularizing, that can go quite far into mitigating concerns," Jacobs says.
"I can't tell you how frequently ladies become concerned on account of the mental changes they're noticing. Frequently, these are transient changes, however, that doesn't detract from the way that they can be startling."

"We can arm ladies with this data," she says.

34 MENOPAUSE SIDE EFFECTS

Menopause and perimenopause can cause a scope of side effects that might shift from one individual to another.

1. Hot glimmers
Hot glimmers are among the most widely recognized side effects of menopause. They make somebody abruptly become hot, sweat-soaked, and flushed, particularly in the face, neck, and chest. Certain individuals likewise experience chills.
Hot glimmers are unexpected sensations of intensity that spread for the most part through the face, neck, and chest. Night sweats happen when hot blazes happen around the evening time. Up to 85 percent of ladies report hot blazes during menopause.

Peruse on to look into the reasons for hot glimmers and night sweats and how you can treat them at home or with medicine.
As indicated by certain appraisals, the event of hot blazes might run for a normal of 5.2 years. What's more, the previous in life they happen, the more drawn out period they might endure.

Hot glimmers and night sweats happen previously and during menopause in light of changing chemical levels, including estrogen and progesterone, influencing the internal heat level's control.

Changes in these chemical levels influence the activity of different chemicals that are liable for directing the internal heat levels. This causes the trademark sensations of abrupt warmth, flushing, and exorbitant perspiring.

The recurrence of hot blazes and night sweats contrasts between individuals. Some mainly experience periodic hot blazes while, for other people, the side effects can impede day-to-day existence.

Treatment and counteraction
Although a few ladies figure out how to manage menopause-related hot blazes and night sweats and can carry on with an ordinary existence with them, for different ladies they can be very upset.

Specialists prescribe that individuals use way of life changes to oversee hot glimmers for quite a long time before attempting drugs.

Individuals can attempt the accompanying techniques to diminish or forestall menopausal hot glimmers and night sweats:

Home solutions for hot glimmers and night sweats
Individuals can embrace a progression of basic way of life changes to adapt to menopausal hot glimmers.

Various elements might increment hot glimmers and night sweats in various individuals. People can have a go at making a note of triggers and keeping away from them. As per the Public Organization of Maturing, normal triggers include:

liquor
zesty food
caffeine
smoking
Other way-of-life tips include:

Remain cool. Wear light garments or dress in layers so you can eliminate them when a hot glimmer strikes.
Keep a fan close to the bed. This will help when individuals experience night sweats.
Keep the room temperature low. Open windows and utilize a fan or forced air system to keep air circling in the room.
Clean up during the day and before bed.
Run cool water over the wrists. There are many veins in the wrists, so this might be an effective method for chilling rapidly.
Keep a sound weight. Hot blazes can be more incessant and serious assuming that individuals are overweight or fat. Keep a sound load by doing customary activities and having a functioning way of life.
Unwind and diminish pressure. Slow and profound breathing and contemplation are strategies that can

assist with easing pressure and decreasing hot flashes. Alternative prescriptions
Many individuals find help from the side effects of menopause through utilizing elective medication rehearses, however, these cures may not work for everybody.

Psyche and body procedures that might further develop side effects include:

Care reflection. Research from 2011 proposes that care might decrease how much annoyance ladies experience from hot glimmers and night sweats.
Mental social treatment (CBT). Research from 2014 recommends that CBT can decrease how
 dangerous individuals find hot glimmers and night sweats.
Dietary enhancements
Certain individuals might find that homegrown cures help. Be that as it may, there is little exploration about their adequacy, and some might interface with different meds or make destructive side impacts.

If individuals wish to attempt dietary enhancements to work on hot blazes, they can get some information about the accompanying:

Phytoestrogens. A survey of studies from 2015 recommends that phytoestrogens may decrease the recurrence of hot glimmers without making serious side impacts. Phytoestrogens are plant intensifies that have a few comparable properties to estrogen.

Dark cohosh. Dark cohosh is a homegrown planning. A 2010 survey of studies proposes that this supplement might lessen the recurrence of hot blazes and night sweats.

Medicine

Assuming somebody encounters extreme hot glimmers or night sweats that interfere with their day-to-day routines or cause elevated degrees of pain, a specialist might suggest the accompanying drugs:

Chemical substitution treatment (HRT)

Chemical treatment, or chemical substitution treatment (HRT), is where individuals take a drug that contains estrogen to control chemical levels. HRT can ease numerous menopausal side effects, including hot glimmers and night sweats.

Ladies who had their uterus eliminated by a methodology called hysterectomy can take estrogen alone.

Yet, ladies who have their uterus are in danger of endometrial malignant growth assuming that they do as such, and they ought to take a medicine that contains both estrogen and progesterone. Joining these two chemicals might lessen the gamble of endometrial malignant growth contrasted with directing estrogen alone.

A specialist will tailor chemical treatments for the person, as per significant gamble factors, and will recommend the least compelling portion of chemicals to decrease incidental effects.

Specialists don't typically suggest chemical treatment for ladies who have had a sort of disease that is delicate to chemicals, like bosom malignant growth. The justification for this is that these diseases fill quicker within the sight of extra chemicals. Essentially, specialists don't suggest this treatment for ladies who have had a blood coagulation.

Antidepressants
Energizer drugs can likewise be utilized to decrease hot blazes and night sweats, even though they are not quite so compelling as chemical treatment.

Notwithstanding, they are a decent choice for ladies who can't get chemical treatment.

The FDA endorses the utilization of paroxetine, a stimulant, to treat hot glimmers. Different antidepressants may likewise help, including venlafaxine and fluoxetine.

Wooziness, sickness, dry mouth, weight gain, or sexual brokenness are conceivable results of these prescriptions.

Antidepressants can be a powerful treatment for hot blazes and may be taken during the menopausal change when side effects are happening.
Different prescriptions
Other physician-recommended drugs can be utilized to assuage hot blazes and night sweats. Nonetheless, these are off-mark so not endorsed for this utilization and ought not to be taken for menopausal side effects except if recommended by a specialist. These include:

Clonidine, an enemy of hypertensive medication typically used to bring down hypertension. It very well may be taken as a pill or by skin fix. Conceivable incidental effects incorporate obstruction, wooziness, trouble resting, and dry mouth.
Gabapentin, an enemy of epileptic medication normally used to treat seizures. Conceivable secondary effects are trouble resting, discombobulation, and migraines.
Standpoint
A great many people experience hot glimmers and night sweats while going through menopause.

A few ladies just experience periodic hot glimmers that don't impede day-to-day existence, however for other people, they can be truly awkward.

Individuals can utilize home solutions to assist with menopausal side effects, and in serious cases, they can utilize drugs, including chemical treatments.

It is fitting to converse with a specialist about the best and most secure techniques for easing side effects, as these can shift between people.

2. Night sweats
Night sweats are hot blazes that happen around the evening time. Researchers don't know why they happen, but rather apparently falling estrogen levels can influence the nerve center, which manages internal heat levels.

3. Sporadic periods
All through the menopausal progress, having unpredictable or missed periods is regular. In the long run, an individual will quit having periods totally.

4. Temperament changes
Temperament changes are erratic changes in mindset irrelevant to life-altering situations. They can make somebody feel abruptly miserable, tearful, or irate. Mindset changes are normal during perimenopause and menopause.

5. Bosom touchiness
Bosom delicacy is one more typical side effect of menopause, however, its recurrence will, in general, diminish in the later stages.

6. Diminished charisma
Menopause likewise generally influences moxie — an individual's craving for sex. This can be the immediate

consequence of having lower levels of testosterone and estrogen, which can make actual excitement more troublesome.
Nonetheless, it can likewise be an optional consequence of different side effects of menopause, for example, temperament changes or a symptom of a drug.

7. Vaginal dryness
As female sex chemicals guarantee that there is satisfactory dissemination of blood around the vagina, an absence of them can diminish the bloodstream and, thusly, normal grease. This might cause dryness, which can be awkward or make penetrative sex more troublesome.

8. Cerebral pains
Somebody entering menopause might encounter more continuous cerebral pains or headache episodes because of a dunk in estrogen. This can be like the migraines that a few females experience before a period.
In any case, dissimilar to during a commonplace monthly cycle, chemical levels during perimenopause can vacillate all the more capriciously.

9. Repeating UTIs
Urinary parcel diseases (UTIs) become more normal after menopause. This is undoubtedly because of the drop in estrogen that happens following menopause. This drop makes the vaginal tissues slim, prompting

46

dryness, bothering, and different variables that make it simpler for a UTI to create. UTIs are repetitive if an individual encounters at least three out of 1 little while or more in 6 months or less.
An individual can assist with forestalling UTIs in the following ways:

utilizing probiotics
drinking cranberry juice
taking d-mannose supplements
An individual can examine the treatment and counteraction of UTIs with their medical care proficiency.

10. Consuming mouth
A consuming mouth is one more expected side effect of menopause because of hormonal changes. It might appear as a sensation of consuming, delicacy, shivering, heat, or desensitizing in or around the mouth. This is one more aftereffect of hormonal changes.
The bodily fluid chemicals in the mouth engage in sexual relations chemical receptors, which decline with a decrease in estrogen. This can add to agony and distress.

11. Changes in taste
Certain individuals might see changes in their feeling of taste, with more grounded flavors, during menopause. They may likewise encounter a dry mouth, which can prompt a higher gamble of creating gum sickness or pits.

12. Exhaustion

Exhaustion can be an upsetting and once in a while weakening menopause side effect. This could be the consequence of lower-quality rest because of hot glimmers and night sweats or because of hormonal variances themselves.

13. Skin breakout

Skin breakout is a condition that individuals generally partner with pre-adulthood. Nonetheless, a 2019 paper noticed that it is a developing worry among individuals encountering menopause. This is in all likelihood because of the irregularity of chemicals during and after menopause.

The American Foundation of Dermatology Affiliation (AAD) states that because an individual's skin commonly becomes drier and more slender, normal skin breakout medicines can be excessively cruel. The AAD prescribes the accompanying ways of aiding to treat and forestall menopausal skin inflammation:

Washing the face utilizing an item that contains salicylic corrosive.
Staying away from skin inflammation items that might dry the skin.
Counseling a dermatologist if the skin breaks out is unmanageable.

14. Other stomach-related changes

48

Female sex chemicals impact the microorganisms an individual has in their mouth and gastrointestinal system. This can actually mean that during menopause, stomach verdure changes in structure. People might see changes in their processing or that they respond diversely to specific food sources.

15. Joint torment

Estrogen helps decline irritation and keep the joints greased up. Subsequently, certain individuals experience joint agony because of diminished estrogen. Estrogen is liable for controlling liquid levels all through the body, so when the body turns out to be low in this chemical, females are more inclined to joint throbs or menopausal joint inflammation.

16. Muscle strain and hurts

People encountering perimenopause or menopause can likewise experience muscle strain
or hurt. This is because of similar variables as menopausal joint agony.

17. Electric shock sensations

Certain individuals can encounter impressions that look like electric shocks during perimenopause and menopause. It isn't clear what causes this, yet it could be the consequence of changing chemical levels in the sensory system.

18. Irritation

As estrogen is connected with collagen creation and skin hydration, a decrease in this chemical can prompt expanded irritation or dryness, normally around the vulva, however may likewise happen somewhere else. Get methods for overseeing tingling during menopause.

19. Rest aggravation

A singular's rest can become lighter or disturbed for some reason during menopause. They might wake as often as possible because of night sweats, get up prior, or find it challenging to get to rest.

A sleeping disorder alludes to the trouble of falling or staying unconscious. It is a typical involvement with menopause and may happen because of hormonal changes. After menopause, an individual's ovaries produce a lot of lower measures of specific chemicals, including estrogen and progesterone.

It might likewise be an optional consequence of different side effects of menopause, like hot blazes.

Peruse on for additional data on menopause and sleep deprivation, including why it works out, how long it might endure, and what clinical medicines and integral treatments are available. Yes — a sleeping disorder is an incessant event during perimenopause and menopause. Certain individuals just experience gentle or intermittent rest unsettling influences, however, for other people, the sleep deprivation can be extreme.

As indicated by a 2018 article, 26% of individuals going through perimenopause and menopause experience a sleeping disorder that influences their day-to-day exercises.

In females, the pace of a sleeping disorder increases with age. As per the Investigation of Ladies' Wellbeing, The country over (SWAN), the commonness of rest problems is as per the following:

16-42% in premenopause
39-47% in perimenopause
35-60% in postmenopause
For what reason does menopause cause sleep deprivation?
Research on the specific reason for sleep deprivation during menopause doesn't highlight one clear reason. A few things might add to it, including:

Hormonal changes
Some proof recommends that low chemical levels can improve the probability of sleep deprivation during menopause.

As indicated by the SWAN, past longitudinal examinations have found a connection between lower levels of estradiol and less fortunate rest. This is particularly obvious if the decrease in chemicals happens rapidly, as it does after an individual goes through a medical procedure to eliminate the ovaries.

Hot glimmers

Some of the time, a sleeping disorder occurs during menopause in light of hot blazes or night sweats. These side effects can disturb rest, causing successive waking.

Hot blazes, which are one of the alleged vasomotor side effects, are normal in menopause, influencing 75-85% of individuals going through menopause.
Hot glimmers cause an unexpected feeling of intensity around the face and neck and frequently happen with perspiring and a quick heartbeat.

Decrease in melatonin
Melatonin is a chemical that assumes a key part in the rest wake cycle, assisting keep peopling sleeping. It is particularly significant toward the beginning of rest. Notwithstanding, melatonin levels seem to diminish with age, which might cause rest unsettling influences.

It isn't evident whether there is a connection between menopause and a decrease in melatonin. Some proof recommends that there is and that people during postmenopause have less melatonin than those during premenopause.

Emotional well-being
For some individuals, menopause flags a significant change. It is likewise a sign that an individual is progressing in years. This, alongside the side effects of menopause, can affect a person's psychological well-being.

Numerous emotional well-being conditions, including uneasiness and discouragement, influence rest. Nonetheless, sleep deprivation can likewise make despondency more probable. The connection between rest and state of mind is bidirectional, and changing chemical levels can likewise assume a part.

How long will sleep deprivation endure?
How long sleep deprivation endures during and after menopause relies upon many elements. Each individual who goes through menopause has an alternate encounter. Some will find that the side effects last longer than they accomplish for other people.

An individual's chemical levels can begin to change 7-10 years before an individual's last period. After this point, individuals can keep on having side effects like hot glimmers for a very long time.

Estradiol levels keep on declining for the initial 1-6 years in early postmenopause, which might bring about proceeded with side effects.

It is significant, notwithstanding, that there are medicines and treatments accessible that can diminish rest troubles. It is likewise vital to address whatever other variables that might be adding to unfortunate rest quality.
Clinical medicines for a sleeping disorder during menopause

The primary treatment for menopause-related sleep deprivation is chemical treatment. This works by supplanting the lost chemicals, which can further develop numerous menopause side effects. Individuals might find that they rest better and experience fewer hot blazes while utilizing this treatment.

Chemical treatment is accessible in skin gels, creams, and fixes. Individuals can likewise take it inside through tablets or an embed.

Another potential treatment is a low-portion particular serotonin reuptake inhibitor (SSRI).

Specialists normally recommend SSRIs for emotional well-being conditions, however, these prescriptions can likewise diminish the recurrence of hot glimmers, which might assist with rest. In any case, it is significant that sleep deprivation can likewise happen as a symptom of SSRIs.

For individuals who are encountering temperament changes, nervousness, or melancholy, talk treatment might help them comprehend and adapt to these sentiments. Decreasing the effect of psychological well-being conditions may likewise help rest.

Specialists seldom recommend resting pills to treat a sleeping disorder, as these can have serious side impacts. Many are likewise habit-forming and are not reasonable for dealing with a drawn-out rest issue.

Normal and reciprocal treatments
As indicated by a 2019 survey, no investigation has discovered that homegrown or dietary enhancements reliably assist with menopause side effects. Nonetheless, there are numerous alternate ways individuals can attempt to make rest more straightforward during menopause.

The following are some proof-based approaches:

Keeping away from caffeine, nicotine, and liquor
Smoking, polishing off caffeine, and drinking liquor can all make it more hard to rest. While it might appear to be that liquor makes individuals sluggish, even a limited quantity diminishes general rest quality.

An individual can attempt to lessen or keep away from any of these, particularly in the early evening and night.

Fragrant healing
Fragrant healing might be useful in actuating unwinding and diminishing hot blazes.

In a clinical preliminary including 100 ladies, scientists found that following 12 weeks of lavender natural oil inward breath, the members had half less hot blazes.

Different investigations have additionally found that fragrance-based treatment along with rub was more viable than back rub or fragrant healing without anyone else.

Spellbinding
A 2019 survey takes note that there is proof that spellbinding might decrease the recurrence and seriousness of hot blazes by up to half.

Also, for individuals whose sleeping disorder results from hot glimmers, spellbinding might be a useful reciprocal treatment.

Yoga
A few examinations have found that yoga gainfully affects the mental side effects of menopause. On the off chance that an individual is experiencing issues dozing because of stress or tension, yoga practice might assist with decreasing these side effects.

Be that as it may, the aftereffects of different investigations on yoga have been blended. This is somewhat because there are many styles of yoga and various approaches to rehearsing, which might prompt conflicting outcomes.
Different variables that can add to a sleeping disorder
Many variables, not just those connected with menopause, can add to a sleeping disorder. They include:

stress
an awkward or boisterous rest climate

openness to blue light from screens of electronic gadgets like telephones, televisions, or tablets
awful dreams or night dread
interruption to an individual's circadian musicality because of a sporadic rest plan, fly slack, or shift work
rest problems
Certain drugs can likewise cause sleep deprivation as an incidental effect. As indicated by the AARP, these include:

beta-blockers
corticosteroids
statins
SSRIs
a blend of chondroitin and glucosamine
alpha-blockers
cholinesterase inhibitors
angiotensin II receptor blockers
angiotensin changing over catalyst inhibitors
nonsedating H1 agonists
When to contact a specialist
An individual encountering sleep deprivation ought to look for direction from a specialist if:

they experienced issues dozing for a really long time
Their sleeping disorder is influencing their day-to-day routine and making it hard to adapt
improving their propensities and sleep time routine has not made a difference
A specialist will attempt to figure out the thing that is causing an individual's sleep deprivation and whether

there is a connection to menopause. By running tests, they will want to get a superior feeling of what is adding to the issue and how best to treat it.

In outline

A sleeping disorder is a typical side effect of menopause and gives off an impression of being more pervasive in individuals with lower levels of chemicals like estradiol.

A sleeping disorder in menopause may likewise be more normal in individuals who experience hot glimmers around evening time or who have lower levels of melatonin.

Supplanting lost chemicals with chemical treatment might assist with further developing menopause-related a sleeping disorder. Making changes to an individual's way of life and day-to-day schedule may likewise demonstrate power.

A few integral treatments, like fragrant healing and spellbinding, may diminish hot blazes and the rest interruption that the hot glimmers can cause.

Many elements influence rest, including an individual's rest climate, age, psychological well-being, and certain meds. It is fitting to contact a specialist so they can research the reason for a sleeping disorder.

20. Trouble concentrating

A decrease in estrogen can once in a while cause mental fogginess or trouble concentrating. Hot glimmers and rest issues may likewise be contributing variables.

21. Memory slips

58

Similarly, as with fixation and concentration, menopause can likewise influence memory. Once more, this could be an immediate consequence of lower estrogen levels or compromised rest.

22. Diminishing hair

During menopause, balding or diminishing is one more aftereffect of ovarian hormonal vacillations. This makes the hair follicles contract, implying that hair develops all the more leisurely and sheds seriously easily. Losing hair can trouble. It can essentially affect an individual's satisfaction, here and there prompting side effects like sadness, nervousness, and low confidence.

If an individual is stressed over balding, they might wish to contact a specialist or a dermatologist to examine the reason for their balding and potential medicines.

This article examines what causes going bald during menopause and how shampoos might assist with diminishing going bald and possibly support hair regrowth. It likewise records a scope of shampoos an individual might wish to consider while checking out diminishing hair because of menopause.
What causes going bald during menopause?
Changing estrogen levels in an individual's body might be connected to going bald during different phases of life, including menopause.

Different reasons for going bald during menopause incorporate hereditary qualities, elevated degrees of stress, and a few meds.

Nourishing lacks may likewise cause going bald. A few nutrients and minerals that might impact hair development include:

vitamin D
B nutrients
vitamin A
zinc
selenium
iron

A recent report likewise proposes that low estrogen levels delivered by the ovaries during menopause could cause going bald.

Nonetheless, for the most part, state, there is a requirement for more exploration to affirm the connection between estrogen and balding, particularly during menopause.

Female example going bald is as yet not completely perceived. Commonly, the reason connects with androgen levels. In any case, certain individuals experience female example balding without androgens during menopause. The reason might be hereditary.

An individual ought to talk with a specialist if they experience going bald around menopause, as there are many sorts of females going bald with various potential causes requiring explicit medicines.
What are going bald shampoos?
Going bald shampoos incorporate fixings that might assist with forestalling balding and support hair development. They may likewise contain fixings that work on the general soundness of an individual's hair.

Well-known fixings in balding shampoos include:

Biotin: A little clinical review has shown proof of further hair development in people utilizing items with biotin. Notwithstanding, this study noticed that proof of the viability of biotin for hair development is restricted.
Caffeine: Exploration has proposed that caffeine might be useful in treating balding, yet not many examinations without huge restrictions demonstrate this.
Epigallocatechin-3-gallate (EGCG): Found in green tea, EGCG decreased balding in mice in a more seasoned 2011 review.
How do going bald shampoos function?
Numerous balding shampoos center around working on the state of an individual's scalp to energize hair development.

Research has shown that shampoos that sustain the scalp with cell reinforcements and boundary-improving specialists can diminish shedding and protect hair wellbeing. They may likewise eliminate the overabundance of scalp oil and buildup from the scalp that might obstruct follicles and forestall hair development.

Oxidative weight on the scalp, some of the time brought about by a creature called Malassezia, can add to balding, as indicated by a recent report. The writers state that the state of the scalp can straightforwardly influence hair development and hair maintenance and that shampoos that lessen the presence of Malassezia on the scalp might assist with forestalling going bald.

What to search for in a cleanser for diminishing hair because of menopause
Balding shampoos incorporate explicit fixings as a result of their detailed advantages on hair development and their capacity to lessen going bald.

Research in some cases upholds the advantages of a portion of these fixings.

For instance, a 2020 survey of existing examinations into the viability of herbal concentrate saw palmetto for hair development found that oral and skin saw palmetto might be a successful treatment choice for androgenetic alopecia, or male example balding. In any case, the review noticed that more examination is expected to demonstrate the revealed advantages of saw palmetto.

A few shampoos contain a fixing called phyto-caffeine, which really diminished balding and expanded hair strength in a recent report.

The sex chemical dihydroxy testosterone (DHT) can set off going bald in menopausal individuals. Hormonal changes that happen during menopause can actuate DHT. Therefore, numerous balding shampoos contain DHT blockers that assist with forestalling further balding.

What to search for in a cleanser for diminishing hair because of menopause
Balding shampoos incorporate explicit fixings in light of their detailed advantages on hair development and their capacity to decrease going bald.

Research now and again upholds the advantages of a portion of these fixings.
For instance, a 2020 survey of existing examinations into the viability of herbal concentrate saw palmetto for hair development found that oral and skin saw palmetto might be a successful treatment choice for androgenetic alopecia, or male example going bald. Notwithstanding, the review noticed that more exploration is expected to demonstrate the revealed advantages of saw palmetto.

A few shampoos contain a fixing called phyto-caffeine, which really diminished going bald and expanded hair strength in a recent report.

The sex chemical dihydroxy testosterone (DHT) can set off balding in menopausal individuals. Hormonal changes that happen during menopause can enact DHT. Thus, numerous balding shampoos contain DHT blockers that assist with forestalling further hair loss.
How to utilize going bald shampoos
Individuals who use shampoos to forestall or turn around balding can utilize them consistently, similarly as they would with a cleanser.

Surveys for the overwhelming majority of the items remembered for this article note that it can require 2-3 months so that an individual might be able to get results.

Top shampoos for diminishing hair because of menopause
Kindly note that the essayist of this article has not attempted these items. All data introduced is simply research-based and right at the hour of distribution.

Plantur 39 Phyto-Caffeine Cleanser
Plantur 39 states that this cleanser is for individuals encountering diminishing hair because of menopause. As per the internet-based item depiction, the cleanser contains phyto-caffeine to decrease hair diminishing and zinc to help hair development.
Furthermore, it incorporates niacin to support hair completion and increment supplement stream to hair follicles.
The item costs $18.45 per jug and accompanies a 60-day unconditional promise.

Kérastase Densifique Bain Densité Cleanser
This cleanser utilizes ceramides to shield hair from harm and hyaluronic corrosive to increment hydration.
The maker claims it makes an individual's hair look thicker and better.
The item costs $31.49 for an 8.5 liquid ounce (fl oz) bottle.

Waterman's Hair Development Cleanser
The producer expresses that this cleanser is reasonable for individuals with diminishing hair because of menopause.
It incorporates biotin, caffeine, and argan oil to advance hair development and reinforce existing hair.
The organization likewise asserts that the sulfate-and without paraben cleanser further develops dissemination to the scalp to invigorate hair development.
The cleanser arrives in a set with a jug of conditioner and costs $35.

Bellisso Biotin Cleanser
The maker asserts this cleanser forestalls going bald and fortifies hair at the follicles. Fixings incorporate biotin, hydrolyzed keratin, and supplement thick botanicals.

The cleanser accompanies a jug of conditioner that the producer cases can obstruct DHT.

The cleanser and conditioner set costs $29.99.ThickTails Invigorating Hair Cleanser
ThickTails claims this cleanser blocks DHT and contains a hyper-anagen complex mix of fixings to advance hair development.

Other hair and scalp-sustaining fixings remembered for this item are:

saw palmetto
caffeine
vitamin B5
biotin
The organization guarantees its item is paraben-, sulfate-, and mercilessness-free and reasonable for a variety of treated hair.

The cleanser and conditioner set costs $39.95.Nioxin Framework 4
This cleanser utilizes vex root separate, saw palmetto, niacin, biotin, and B nutrients to unclog hair follicles and advance hair development.

The organization guarantees the item functions admirably on fine and variety-treated hair.

The cleanser arrives in a set with a conditioner and a scalp treatment, which costs $29.99.Alterna Haircare Caviar Hostile to Maturing Clinical Densifying Cleanser

Alterna states that this caviar cleanser purifies the hair delicately and lessens the buildups and DHT that can make hair slim.
The critical fix in this cleanser is caviar removal, which contains omega-3 unsaturated fats that the organization cases can reestablish dampness, and flexibility, and try to please an individual's hair.
An 8.5 fl oz bottle costs $34.

Pura d'Or Unique Gold Name Against Diminishing Biotin Cleanser
This cleanser contains 17 DHT blockers along with nutrients and minerals that the organization cases can support hair development.

Different fixings include:

saw palmetto
pumpkin seed
annoy
tea tree oil
aloe
niacin
A 16 fl oz bottle costs $29.74

Oftentimes clarified pressing issues
Coming up next are normal inquiries and replies about shampoos for diminishing hair during menopause:

How would I stop going bald during menopause?

Hormonal changes during menopause can actuate DHT, which has been connected to going bald. A few shampoos contain biotin, which serves to deactivate and switch the adverse consequences of DHT.

One 2019 investigation discovered that solution medicines containing 2% ketoconazole, typically endorsed for treating dandruff, may further develop going bald.

Powerful medicines, for example, minoxidil are typically utilized close by shampoos and left on the scalp for a more drawn-out period. A specialist can recommend these medicines for use close by over-the-counter shampoos.
Be that as it may, there is no dependable technique for forestalling or switching balding during menopause. A mix of medicines and way of life changes might be important.
Does balding from menopause bounce back?
Balding made by menopause may not be reversible due to the primary changes in the hair follicle brought about by hormonal changes.
Nonetheless, an individual might wish to investigate medicines for menopause-prompted going bald. These incorporate way-of-life changes, like eating a decent eating regimen, practicing consistently, diminishing pressure, and utilizing specific going bald drugs.

In synopsis

Many individuals experience going bald during menopause because of hormonal changes happening inside the body.

Shampoos containing fixings that advance hair development and scalp wellbeing, like caffeine, biotin, and cell reinforcements, may assist an individual with going bald, empowering hair to bounce back or decreasing how much hair they lose.

Normally, skin and oral prescriptions are more useful, or an individual can add them to their cleanser routine. A specialist can endorse medicines or prompt choices.

On the off chance that an individual is stressed over going bald or encountering bothering or different issues with the skin on their scalp close by balding, they might consider reaching a specialist or a dermatologist to look for suitable treatment.

Side effects that might show a hidden condition include consuming, tingling, scaling, redness of the scalp, or bare patches. Individuals with these side effects can visit a dermatologist. The dermatologist can examine other treatment choices or recommend blood tests to preclude thyroid problems, frailty, hemochromatosis, or other potential reasons for balding around menopause.

23. Fragile nails

During or after menopause, the body may not create sufficient keratin, which is the substance that nails need for areas of strength to remain. This can prompt fragile, powerless nails that break or break without any problem.

24. Weight gain

People can put on weight because of a few variables during menopause. A decrease in estrogen can bring about weight gain, as can bring down measures of actual work. Mind-set changes can likewise imply that a female eats uniquely in contrast to normal.

25. Stress incontinence

Stress incontinence alludes to a successive or unexpected desire to pee. Certain individuals additionally allude to it as an "overactive bladder." This side effect is normal during menopause, as changes in chemical levels can make the bladder and pelvic muscles become more fragile.

26. Mixed-up spells

Hormonal changes in menopause can cause nervousness. A recent report expressed that tipsiness is one of the most widely recognized side effects of menopause, yet the specific reason for it isn't known. In any case, the review directed at 470 people found that dazedness in menopause might have an association with uneasiness.

27. Sensitivities

A few females demolish sensitivity side effects when they experience menopause. This happens because, during menopause, females can have spikes in receptors. The fact that causes hypersensitive responses makes the receptor the compound.

28. Osteoporosis

During perimenopause, a decrease in estrogen can likewise bring about a deficiency of bone thickness. In extreme cases, this can prompt osteoporosis, which makes the bones more delicate and break without any problem.

29. Sporadic heartbeat

Certain individuals might encounter a sporadic heartbeat or palpitations during or after menopause. It is dependably smart to examine side effects connecting with the heart with a medical services proficient.

30. Tinnitus

Tinnitus is a side effect that includes hearing a sound that has no outside cause. This can be remembered as a ringing for the ears, thundering, or humming. It might influence one or two ears. Different indications of tinnitus might include:

whistling
murmuring
clicking
murmuring
screeching

While the specific predominance is obscure, a recent report has shown that individuals going through menopause might encounter tinnitus. This might be because of the hormonal changes inside the body. This examination has additionally shown that hormonal substitution treatment (HRT) may assist with treating tinnitus.

31. Crabbiness

Either because of hormonal vacillations or the impact of other menopause side effects, individuals encountering this change might feel peevish. Stress or an absence of rest may likewise add to this.

32. Sorrow

For certain individuals, hormonal irregular characteristics might set off gloom. An absence of rest and stress can add to this.

At times, menopause might set off sorrow or low temperament because of the change it connotes in a female's life. Any huge life-altering event can assume a part in sadness, regardless of whether the change is a positive one.

33. Nervousness

Nervousness is another temperament-related side effect that certain individuals experience during menopause. It might deteriorate around evening time or just happen discontinuously as chemical levels vacillate.

Both menopause-related gloom and nervousness might be situational and improve once chemicals level out.

34. Alarm jumble

Now and again, people might encounter fits of anxiety during menopause. At the point when these assaults happen out of the blue or out of nowhere, they can show alarm jumble. This might occur because of hormonal changes or the apprehension about feeling restless itself.

During a fit of anxiety, an individual might encounter overpowering feelings, including weakness and dread. Actual side effects can incorporate a quick heartbeat, fast breathing, perspiring, and shaking.

Fits of anxiety frequently occur in unambiguous circumstances that trigger elevated pressure. In any case, certain individuals experience them over and again, with no reasonable triggers. In this situation, the individual might have an alarm jumble.

A specialist will utilize measures from the Symptomatic and Factual Manual of Mental Issues, Fifth Version (DSM-5) to analyze alarm jumble.

Around 1 of every 75 individuals have alarm jumble, as indicated by the American Mental Affiliation (APA). It can seriously impact personal satisfaction. Notwithstanding, fits of anxiety and frenzy problems are both emotional well-being issues that medicines can help make due.
A fit of anxiety might be a secluded issue or a repeating side effect of a frenzy problem.
In any case, an assault can be terrifying, disturbing, and awkward. The sentiments are more extreme than those of stress that individuals normally experience.

Fits of anxiety ordinarily last 5-20 minutes, however, the side effects can wait for as long as 60 minutes.
As per the Nervousness and Melancholy Relationship of America, a fit of anxiety includes something like four of the accompanying side effects:

chest torment and uneasiness
chills or feeling hot
tipsiness and unsteadiness
a feeling of dread toward biting the dust
a feeling of dread toward letting completely go or "going off the deep end"
heart palpitations, a sporadic heartbeat, or a fast pulse
deadness or shivering
shaking, perspiring, or shudder
inconvenience breathing, which might cause to gag
feeling isolated from the real world
sickness and a resentful stomach
Individuals with fits of anxiety at times foster agoraphobia, which includes a feeling of dread toward circumstances where help or a departure might be challenging to get to.

The side effects of a fit of anxiety can look like those of other ailments, including lung issues, heart conditions, or thyroid issues.
Once in a while, an individual having a fit of anxiety looks for crisis clinical consideration since they feel as though they are having a coronary failure. Here, figure out how to differentiate.

What is alarm jumble?
Alarm jumble is a psychological wellness condition, and fits of anxiety are a side effect.

Many individuals experience no less than one fit of anxiety sooner or later, yet individuals with alarm jumble experience repetitive assaults.

The side effects regularly emerge in early adulthood, around the ages of 18-25 years, yet alarm turmoil can be fostered in kids. Happening in females as males is two times as reasonable.

Hereditary and natural variables might improve the probability of having an alarm jumble, yet researchers presently can't seem to recognize a connection with a particular quality or synthetic.

The issue might arise when an individual with specific hereditary highlights faces natural burdens. These incorporate significant life-altering events, for example, having a first child or venturing out from home. A background marked by physical or sexual maltreatment may likewise build the gamble.

Alarm turmoil might be created when an individual who has encountered a few fits of anxiety becomes terrified of having another. This dread can make them pull out from loved ones and forgo heading outside or visiting spots where a fit of anxiety might happen.

Alarm turmoil can seriously restrict an individual's personal satisfaction, however compelling medicines are accessible.

Causes

Uneasiness is a characteristic reaction to stretch, yet if nervousness levels become too high, this can prompt a frenzy.

At the point when the mind gets admonitions of risk, it makes the adrenal organ aware of the delivery of adrenaline, which is some of the time called epinephrine or the "survival" chemical.

A surge of adrenaline can stimulate the heartbeat and raise circulatory strain and the pace of relaxing. These are qualities of a fit of anxiety.

Might you at any point pass on from a fit of anxiety?

Risk factors

Various issues can improve the probability of having fits of anxiety and frenzy problems. These include:

hereditary variables

significant pressure or life changes

caffeine, tobacco, liquor, sporting medications, and sweet food sources and beverages

Likewise, fits of anxiety can be a side effect of different circumstances, for example,

summed up nervousness jumble

fanatical urgent problem

post-horrendous pressure problem

Finding

Involving the rules in the DSM-5, a specialist might analyze alarm jumble on the off chance that the individual has:

regular, startling fits of anxiety
had a continuous feeling of dread toward having a fit of anxiety for no less than a month
altogether changed their way of behaving because of this trepidation
no other condition, like social fear, and no utilization of meds or medications that could represent the side effects.

Treatment
The most widely recognized medicines for alarm jumble are prescriptions and psychotherapy.
As indicated by the APA, many individuals feel significantly improved when they comprehend what the frenzy problem is — and the way that normal it is.
An individual might profit from mental social treatment, in some cases abbreviated to CBT. It can assist them with recognizing triggers and better approaches for confronting tough spots.
Another choice is interoceptive openness, which trains an individual to become used to the side effects of a fit of anxiety in a protected climate. The point is to diminish the apprehension about an assault and to separate the side effects into sensible stages.
In the interim, unwinding procedures, for example, slow breathing and perception can likewise help.

For certain individuals, a specialist may likewise endorse at least one of the accompanying medications:

Benzodiazepines: These can treat side effects of uneasiness, and models incorporate alprazolam (Xanax) and clonazepam (Klonopin).
Specific serotonin reuptake inhibitors (SSRIs): These are regularly used to treat discouragement, and a few models incorporate fluoxetine (Prozac), paroxetine. (Paxil), and sertraline (Zoloft).
Serotonin and norepinephrine reuptake inhibitors (SNRIs): These are additional antidepressants, and one model is venlafaxine hydrochloride (Effexor XR).
Beta-blockers: These can manage the heartbeat.
SSRIs and SNRIs are long-haul medicines and can require a little while to make a difference.
Benzodiazepines can decrease side effects all the more rapidly, yet there is a gamble of reliance.
A few meds produce unfavorable outcomes. It is vital that a specialist works with the individual to track down the most ideal treatment.
In 2020, the Food and Medication Organization (FDA) fortified their admonition about benzodiazepines.
Utilizing these medications can prompt actual reliance, and withdrawal can life-compromise. Consolidating them with liquor, narcotics, and different substances can bring about death. It is fundamental to adhere to the specialist's guidelines while utilizing these medications.
Counteraction
Different tips can assist with decreasing the recurrence and effect of fits of anxiety.

At the point when a fit of anxiety begins:
Do whatever it takes not to battle it.
Remain where you are.
Practice slow, profound relaxing.
Attempt to envision positive pictures.
Recall that it will before long pass and that isn't
dangerous.
To decrease the gamble of additional assaults:
Find out about fits of anxiety and converse with others
about the experience.
Keep away from substances that can add to the issue,
including caffeine, tobacco, liquor, sporting medications,
and sweet food varieties and beverages.
Get standard rest and exercise to diminish pressure.
Practice yoga, profound breathing, positive perception,
and different strategies for unwinding.
Track down additional procedures here.

Confusions
Without treatment, alarm turmoil can hurt numerous
parts of an individual's life. It might, for instance, lead to:
an unfortunate utilization of liquor, tobacco, or different
substances
fears, like agoraphobia
issues with the everyday schedule
social withdrawal
other well-being concerns, which re
quire continuous clinical consideration
monetary challenges
self-destructive considerations or ways of behaving

Viewpoint
Fits of anxiety and frenzy problems influence many
individuals. The assaults can be startling, however,
there are powerful medicines.
Anybody with worries about fits of anxiety or frenzy
issues ought to get clinical consideration. Getting this
care right off the bat can hold the side effects back from
deteriorating and forestall confusion.

FOUR MENOPAUSE STAGES

lady's conceptive well-being goes through many shifts
over the direction of her lifetime. From the principal
feminine period, through the childbearing years, and the
entire way to menopause and then some, chemicals are
going through significant movements, making each
stage particular. Generally speaking, the pattern of
ladies' well-being can be separated into four
fundamental stages.

Pre-Menopause Stage
During the pre-menopause phase of life, a lady is having
her standard feminine cycle, is thriving in childbearing
years, and has no observable side effects of
menopause. A lady is in the pre-menopause stage
anytime prior to entering perimenopause.

Perimenopause Stage
Perimenopause is a temporary stage between pre-
menopause and menopause. This stage commonly

starts in a lady's 40s and goes on for a long time. During this time, the consequences of hormonal movements will become recognizable as the ovaries gradually quit working. As estrogen creation eases back and fewer eggs are delivered, normal perimenopause side effects, for example, the accompanying frequently happen:

More limited and progressively unpredictable periods
Successive changes in the state of mind
Diminished sex drive
Hot blazes and night sweats
Vaginal dryness
Cerebral pains
Mind haze or trouble concentrating
Hurting joints or muscles
While fruitfulness is diminished and generation more outlandish, a lady can in any case become pregnant during perimenopause.

Menopause Stage
Menopause can influence ladies going from their 30s to their 60s. Nonetheless, the normal period of menopause beginning in American ladies is 51. To be viewed as in menopause, a lady must have had a feminine cycle for 12 successive months. The ovaries have quit working completely and are done delivering eggs.

For menopausal ladies, hot blazes are the most well-known grumbling. Moreover, these hot glimmers might be joined by an expanded pulse. Ladies may likewise see diminished bosom completion, more slender hair, expanded development of beard growth, or urinary incontinence as the pelvic floor turns out to be looser.

Post-Menopause Stage

When a lady has outperformed an entire year without a feminine cycle, she is viewed as postmenopausal. She will stay in this stage until the end of her life. Luckily, during this time, the side effects that denoted the perimenopause and menopause years started to die down, leaving most ladies all the more truly agreeable. In any case, because of diminished estrogen, the gamble for ailments, for example, osteoporosis and coronary illness increments during this time. For ladies who have arrived at the postmenopausal phase of life, a solid way of life and chemical substitution treatment can be vital to keeping chemical-related complexities under control.

INDIA MENOPAUSE

Because of ovarian deficiency, a few ladies accomplish menopause at an early age because of the way of life factors and hormonal irregular characteristics. Menopause happening before the age of 40 is untimely and somewhere in the range of 40 and 44 years age is right on time, since the normal period of menopause lies somewhere in the range of 45 and 50. The review assessed the pervasiveness of both untimely and early menopause and analyzed the potential related factors that could set off its event in India. The Public Family Wellbeing Review, directed during 2019-2021, was utilized to satisfy the review objective. The review test was isolated into two sections, with age bunch 15-39 and 40-44 for assessing untimely and early menopause, individually. The cox-relative peril model was utilized for the multivariate investigation. The assessed pervasiveness of untimely menopause is 2.2% and early menopause is 16.2%. Lower instructive level, poor monetary condition, smoking, seared food utilization, and early age at menarche are a portion of the huge logical variables. In India, both the extent and without a doubt, the quantity of post-menopausal ladies are developing, consequently it is basic to patch up open conceptive medical services offices to remember menopausal wellbeing fragment for ladies' wellbeing too. Future itemized miniature examinations would help in better comprehension of untimely or early menopausal cases.

The occasion of ovarian disappointment is named menopause. Larger part ladies ordinarily achieve menopause in the age section of 45 and 551. As per the World Wellbeing Association (WHO), regular menopause is characterized as a "super durable suspension of the monthly cycle coming about because of the deficiency of ovarian follicular action", which is ordinarily perceived following a drawn-out sequential amenorrhea2. This is a fundamental physical and hormonal occasion in a solid lady's regenerative cycle. With expanding age, the ovarian capability drains and diminishes its creation of estrogen and progesterone chemicals, and accordingly the progressive decrease in fecundity3,4. So essentially, menopause is the progress of a lady's life from a regenerative stage to a non-conceptive stage, which has organic, profound, sociocultural significance5.

The age circulation of menopause resembles a Gaussian bend going from age 40 to 54, however, the general grouping is around 45-556. A few ladies, because of ovarian deficiency accomplish menopause at an early age because of the way of life factors and hormonal irregular characteristics. Menopause happening before the age of 40 is untimely and somewhere in the range of 40 and 44 years age is right on time, since the regular period of menopause lies somewhere in the range of 45 and 50. The end of menses is set apart by amenorrhea, ascend in gonadotrophin levels, and estrogen deficiency7,8.

As indicated by a Container India concentrate by Ahuja (2016), there are major areas of strength between the beginning stage of menopause and different factors, for example, lack of education, poor financial foundation, underweight, equality, and age at pregnancy9. Studies have shown that age at menarche, breastfeeding of past kids, and age at first pregnancy, assume a vital part in deciding the beginning of menopause10. There are likewise impacts of nulliparity, use of oral preventative pills, having a live birth or not, on the beginning of normal menopause11,12. Menopausal age is related to various variables with incorporate smoking13,14, level of education15, working status16, abortion17, weight index16, and food habits18. Smoking explicitly antagonistically affects regenerative wellbeing and weighty smokers were seen to arrive at menopause earlier19,20, accordingly making it critical to concentrate on its affiliation. Tobacco utilization estrogenically affects the female body which can prompt estrogen capability resistance20. There has not been any steady relationship between the beginning of menopause and the above-expressed factors.

In the next few decades, both the extent and number of Indian ladies aged 45 and past are supposed to forcefully rise. In India, there were around 96 million ladies who were 45 years old or more seasoned as of the 2011 enumeration, and this figure is projected to ascend to 401 million by 202621. By and large, burn through 30 years in the postmenopausal phase of life because the typical future at age 45 is 30 years. The post-menopausal populace might give critical issues to the arrangement of public medical services in the future because of the well-being concerns related to these years, including hypertension, coronary illness, osteoporosis, and a disintegration in the general nature of life22,23. Expanding urbanization and changing ways of life present more prominent difficulties to general well-being. Distinguishing factors related to early menopause are important. The age at menopause is related to the gamble of a few persistent sicknesses like cardiovascular infections, bosom and endometrial diseases, and osteoporosis24,25,26,27. Albeit this issue is disregarded in India, untimely or early menopause has various short- and long-haul negative well-being results. Medical conditions connected with beginning-stage menopause are not notable in India because the determinants and pervasiveness of untimely menopause are not irrefutable, and accordingly comes our significant examination question in regards to something similar.

The speculation is, to test.

H0

There is no massive impact of financial, segment, clinical, and way of life conduct on untimely and beginning stage of menopause against

H1

There is a massive impact of financial, segment, clinical, and way of life conduct on untimely and beginning stages of menopause.

In this way, the review plans to assess the predominance of both untimely and early menopause and analyze the expected related factors in India.

INFORMATION AND STRATEGIES

Information source

The review uses the most recent round of Public Family Wellbeing Overview, directed during 2019-2021. The initial (1993-1993), second (1998-1999), third (2005-2006), fourth (2015-2016) and fifth (2019-2021) round of Public Family Wellbeing Review (NFHS) for investigating the general pattern and the new round until the end of the review. The Public Family Wellbeing Overview (NFHS) is a huge scope, multi-round review led by delegate tests of families all through India. The NFHS is a cooperative task of the Global Foundation for Populace Sciences (IIPS), Mumbai, India; ORC Full scale, Calverton, Maryland, USA and the East-West focus, Honolulu, Hawaii, USA. The Service of Wellbeing and Family Government Assistance (MoHFW), Administration of India, assigned IIPS as a nodal organization, answerable for giving coordination and specialized direction to the NFHS. The fifth round of NFHS was led in 2019-2021, with the interference of

Coronavirus in the middle between. The review was completed for 707 locales, as of 31st Walk 2017. Because of the pandemic lockdown, the hands-on work was in two stages Stage I covered 17 states and association regions from seventeenth June 2019 to 30th January 2020; and Stage II covered 11 states and association domains from second January 2020 to 30th April 2021. 17 field offices gathered data from 636,699 families, 724,115 ladies, and 101,839 men28.

The pregnant ladies and lactating moms during the hour of overview are barred from the examination. Ladies who had gone through a hysterectomy, that is to say, are additionally prohibited from having careful menopause. Two separate datasets are made for the investigation and the example sizes for examination of untimely menopause are 429,446 (ages 15-39), and early menopause 79,643 (ages 40-44).

The review assessed the pervasiveness of untimely and early menopause, and further dissected its deciding variables, using an enormous scope public populace overview. Past examinations in light of NFHS or other public overviews generally included ladies who went through careful menopause as well31,32,33, but this study prohibited it to stay away from misjudgment of the predominance rates for untimely and early menopause, with the perplexing impact of a huge number of hysterectomies. The assessed predominance of untimely menopause is 2.2% and early menopause is 16.2%. A review by 34 had assessed untimely menopause to be 1.5% involving the DLHS 2007-2008 information in India. One more review given the US and Korean populace too processed the predominance of untimely menopause, as 1.7% and 2.8%, separately, and early menopause as 3.4% and 7.2% in US and Korea, respectively35. Notwithstanding, none of the examinations had barred the pregnant and lactating moms from the example, which was viewed in the current review, hence making the ongoing assessment more powerful.

Generally speaking, the review's financial, family arranging, and segment attributes were considerably connected to untimely and early menopause. Ladies in provincial settings are almost certain than those in metropolitan regions to have untimely menopause since they are less inclined to approach medical care services36. The level of training is a huge logical considering untimely and early menopause. Untimely and early menopause rates expanded among ladies with lower levels of training, This outcome is by different examinations as well16,37. As per the current review, ladies from less fortunate families were bound to go through untimely and early menopause, which is predictable with prior examinations in India or other regions15,18. There is a potential neediness and sustenance connected in such a manner. This peculiarity could be made sense of in the manner that ladies in country regions in more unfortunate families, and having less or no schooling have an absence of mindfulness combined with detachment of medical care administrations and poor wholesome eating routine. The diversity of private, financial, and instructive weaknesses has intensified impact that might prompt the beginning stage of menopause.

Way of life decisions, for example, tobacco, liquor, and low-quality food utilization were seen to be contributing variables towards untimely and early menopause. Tobacco smoking during the conceptive cycle or overall smoking had been viewed as a huge component causing untimely menopause 32. The gamble was viewed as relatively higher among female cigarette smokers than the ones who quit smoking. By bringing down the progression of estrogen, tobacco's enemy of estrogen activities accelerates the beginning of menopause 38. In general, this compromises the average hormonal equilibrium in ladies, which affects the whole framework. While smoking is joined with early menopause, the hormonal uneven characteristics bring about rest issues, burdensome side effects, and ultimately weakened mental performance20,39,40. Meat and liquor utilization and actual idleness were freely found to have a huge relationship with untimely menopause in past studies41,42. Dietary examples and the healthful status of a lady had been likewise observed to be contributing elements to untimely menopause. This chance is higher among ladies with low weight records (BMI) or malnourished which is likewise seen from the review results43,44. Fat tissue is where estrogen is put away, and incredibly dainty ladies have lower stores of estrogen, which are all the more effectively depleted. Ladies with higher BMIs have higher measures of estrone (E1) and estradiol (E2) in their bodies, which can postpone menopause. BMI is a vital figure in deciding endogenous estrogen levels45. However, the study demonstrated untimely menopause to be higher among overweight/fat ladies, while early menopause was higher among underweight ladies.

Early age at menarche whenever found to have a huge relationship with untimely and early menopause. A concentrate by Mishra et al. (2017), detailed that ladies who had menarche before the age of 13, had twofold the gamble of encountering untimely menopause and 31% higher gamble of early menopause46. Early menarche has been connected to poor conceptive working, including sporadic periods47,48, PCOS49, and a somewhat higher gamble of endometriosis50, as per prior investigations. Despite past studies46,48 that detailed the nulliparous ladies had a higher possibility of encountering the beginning stage of menopause, the current review showed no critical affiliation. The age at first birth is another inferable component, which shows that untimely and early menopause is higher among the ones whose age at first birth is lower than 18 years33. Ladies who don't become pregnant regularly have a previous menopause than the people who have kids. Furthermore, it is the case that normal elements — going from hereditary qualities to youth natural variables like corpulence, mental pressure, and social climate — may make sense of the affiliation and affect menopause, the date of the principal time frame, and fertility46.

Curiously the utilization of hormonal contraceptives, for example, injectables, pills, and crisis contraception likewise arose as an informative variable for untimely and early menopause. However, there have been concentrates before that expressed the people who utilized oral contraception had encountered untimely menopause less51,52,53. History of end of pregnancy showed a relationship with untimely and early menopause, but not laid out a lot in prior examinations. As well as hurting the uterus, early termination can bring about ovarian brokenness, which can prompt the disappointment of the ovaries. Ready to deliver eggs of normal, ordinary quality. Chemical creation volume can likewise be affected. Moreover, ovarian contamination or obstructed fallopian cylinders might result from hazardous or continuous early termination, and full ovary evacuation, which damages and ages the ovaries54.

Another intriguing outcome is that of the relationship between higher glucose levels with untimely and early menopause. Ladies who have either type 1 diabetes (before age 30) or type 2 diabetes (somewhere in the range of 30 and 39 years) are more likely than indistinguishable ladies without diabetes to encounter menopause prior throughout everyday life. There may be an association between diabetes and changes in the body, regenerative framework, and maturing and working of the ovaries55. Future investigations are expected to decide the possible reasons for the relationship between diabetes and untimely or early menopause. The review gives a pattern for doing future exploration in India by thinking about additional elements and directing causal derivations.

Qualities and restrictions

The review has a few qualities inferable from its public representativeness and systemic vigor. The investigation depends on a public-level populace study that covered a huge scope of information on ladies' well-being that assisted with evaluating the most extreme elements influencing early age at menopause. It was likewise conceivable to reject the ones who had gone through hysterectomy similarly as with the medical procedure done these ladies have lower estrogen levels than different ladies who have achieved untimely or early menopause naturally56. This investigation controlled for the greater part of the elements that could jumble the outcomes.

The review has a few restrictions inferable from the cross-sectional nature. There are chances of reviewing the inclination of the date of the last feminine cycle since it is self-detailed. The way that the ongoing review utilized information from ladies between the ages of 15 and 49 was an unmistakable limitation. To move past this limitation, we utilized endurance models in our examination. These models work best with information that is 'time to occasion information' and that contains blue-penciled cases. Since the review has examined auxiliary information, more point-by-point miniature examinations would help in better comprehension of the untimely or early menopausal cases.

End

The large number of ladies accomplishing menopause at more youthful ages involves concern. This study is a significant commitment to writing that gives a vigorous pervasiveness gauge to untimely and early menopause and comprehensively investigates conceivable logical variables utilizing an enormous scope of public information. Oppressed ladies must approach the legitimate eating regimen and medical services measures because early menopause is related to osteoporosis and other medical issues. To additionally comprehend the connections between broad undernutrition welcomed on by neediness and explicit micronutrient inadequacies that might affect ovarian hold, for example, vitamin D lack, more examination is required. In India, both the extent and without a doubt, the quantity of post-menopausal ladies are developing, consequently it's basic to patch up open conceptive medical services offices to incorporate the right sorts of therapy for them.

The ongoing medical services framework faces trouble in giving satisfactory consideration to the numerous ladies who experience early menopause. The requests of ladies going through early menopause ought to be considered by the taxpayer-supported initiatives currently set up that are intended to address the issues of childbearing ladies. Ladies who are moving toward menopause need help with dealing with the side effects welcomed by hormonal shifts and the menopausal change. Ladies might persevere through vasomotor side effects, urinogenital issues, and mental issues during this time. These ladies might have the option to adapt to the uneasiness they experience with the backing of the treatment and guidance that medical services experts can offer. It is feasible to train medical care experts to offer the necessary guidance and exhortation to manage the issues faced by menopausal ladies; these activities are minimal expense and easy to integrate into current projects. One more technique to support ladies going through untimely menopause to search out the proper clinical consideration is to raise public information on the impeding impacts of untimely menopause on well-being and the meaning of doing so. It is proposed to guarantee medical care admittance to oppressed ladies has been upheld by the information in abundance record, social and segment qualities, and way of life propensities, and there is a desperate need to grow medical care administrations and accordingly the monetary allotments.

WHICH CHEMICALS TO CHECK

Ladies ordinarily notice the signs and side effects of menopause without a conventional determination from their medical services supplier. An adjustment of feminine examples and the presence of hot blazes are typically the principal signs.

Despite the fact that blood tests are not needed, medical services suppliers can run blood or pee tests to decide levels of the chemicals estradiol, follicle-animating chemical (FSH), and luteinizing chemical (LH).[1,2] At menopause, the ovaries become less receptive to FSH and LH chemicals, so the body makes a greater amount of these chemicals to redress. Estradiol and different chemicals decline around menopause too. A medical care supplier can utilize the test results to let know if a lady is in menopause.

During and after menopause, a lady ought to get normal physical, pelvic, bosom, colorectal, and skin tests to screen her well-being.

Your PCP might arrange a blood test to check your degrees of follicle-invigorating chemical (FSH) and estrogen. During menopause, your FSH levels increment and your estrogen levels decline.

During the main portion of your feminine cycle, FSH, a chemical delivered by the foremost pituitary organ, invigorates the development of eggs as well as the creation of a chemical called estradiol.

Estradiol is a type of estrogen that is liable for (in addition to other things) controlling the monthly cycle and supporting the female regenerative plot.

As well as affirming menopause, this blood test can recognize indications of specific pituitary problems. Your PCP might arrange an extra blood test to look at your thyroid-invigorating chemical (TSH), as hypothyroidism can cause side effects that are like menopause.

An as-late supported demonstrative test called the PicoAMH Elisa test estimates how many enemies of Mullerian chemical (AMH) are in the blood. It can assist your primary care physician with deciding when you will enter menopause if you haven't as of now.

EARLY MENOPAUSE

Early menopause will be menopause that starts between the ages of 40 and 45. Untimely menopause begins considerably prior, before age 40. Assuming you begin seeing side effects of menopause before you turn 40, you might be encountering untimely menopause. Early or untimely menopause can occur for various reasons, including:

chromosomal deformities, like Turner Disorder
immune system infections, like thyroid illness
careful expulsion of the ovaries (oophorectomy) or uterus (hysterectomy)
chemotherapy or other radiation treatments for disease
If you're under 40 and haven't had a period in more than 90 days, see your PCP to get tried for early menopause or other fundamental causes.
Your PCP will utilize large numbers of similar tests referenced above for menopause, particularly test
s used to decide your degrees of estrogen and FSH.
Early menopause can expand your gamble for osteoporosis, coronary illness, and other medical issues.
Assuming you suspect that you may be encountering it, getting tried for menopause can assist you with concluding right off the bat how best to deal with your well-being and side effects on the off chance that you've analyzed.
The following analysis
Whenever menopause has been affirmed, your primary care physician will examine treatment choices. You may not require any treatment on the off chance that your side effects aren't serious.

In any case, your primary care physician might prescribe specific meds and chemical treatments to manage side effects that can influence your satisfaction. They may likewise suggest chemical medicines assuming you are more youthful when you arrive at menopause.

A few side effects can make it hard to go about day-to-day exercises, like rest, sex, and unwinding. Be that as it may, you can make the way of life changes to assist with dealing with your side effects:

For hot blazes, hydrate or pass on a space to someplace that is cooler.

Use water-based greases during sex to limit the uneasiness of vaginal dryness.

Eat a nutritious eating routine, and converse with your PCP about taking enhancements to ensure you're getting an adequate number of supplements and nutrients.

Get a lot of ordinary activity, which can assist with deferring the beginning of conditions that occur as you progress in years.

Stay away from caffeine, smoking, and cocktails however much as could be expected. These can cause hot blazes or make it hard to rest.

Get a lot of rest. The quantity of hours fundamental for a decent rest changes from one individual to another, yet seven to nine hours of the night is normally suggested for grown-ups.

Buy water-based ointments on the web.

Menopause can expand your gamble of different circumstances, particularly those related to maturing.

Keep on seeing your PCP for preventive consideration, including ordinary check-ups and actual tests, to ensure that you're mindful of any circumstances and to guarantee your ideal well-being as you age.

WHAT TRIGGERS EARLY MENOPAUSE

What are the side effects of early menopause?
Early menopause can start when you begin having
sporadic periods or periods that are perceptibly longer
or more limited than your normal cycle.

Different side effects of early menopause include:

weighty dying
spotting
periods that last longer than seven days
a more drawn-out measure of time in between periods
In these cases, contact your PCP to check for whatever
other issues that may be causing these side effects.

Other normal side effects of menopause include:

temperament swings
changes in sexual sentiments or want
vaginal dryness
inconvenience dozing
hot glimmers
night sweats
loss of bladder control
What causes early menopause?
There are a few known reasons for early menopause,
however once in a while, the reason is not set in stone.

Hereditary qualities

Assuming there's not an obvious explanation for early menopause, the reason is logically hereditary. Your age at menopause beginning is reasonably acquired.

Knowing when your parent began menopause can give pieces of information about when you'll begin your own. If your parent began menopause early, you're more likely than normal to do likewise.

Notwithstanding, qualities recount just a portion of the story.

Way of life factors
Some way of life variables might affect when you start menopause. Smoking influences estrogen and can add to early menopause.

Some exploration proposes that long-haul or normal smokers are probably going to encounter menopause sooner. Ladies who smoke might begin menopause 1 to 2 years sooner than ladies who don't smoke.
Weight list (BMI) can likewise factor into early menopause. Estrogen is put away in fat tissue. Extremely slight ladies have less estrogen stores, which can be exhausted sooner.

Some exploration likewise recommends that a veggie lover diet, absence of activity, and absence of sun openness all through your life can all cause a beginning stage of menopause.

Chromosome issues

A few chromosomal issues can prompt early menopause. For instance, Turner's condition (additionally called monosomy X and gonadal dysgenesis) includes being brought into the world with a deficient chromosome.

Ladies with Turner disorder have ovaries that don't work true to form. This frequently makes them enter menopause rashly.

Other chromosomal issues can cause early menopause, as well. This incorporates unadulterated gonadal dysgenesis, a minor departure from Turner disorder.

In this condition, the ovaries don't work. All things considered, periods and optional sex attributes should be achieved by chemical substitution treatment, typically during puberty.

Ladies with Delicate X condition, or who are hereditary transporters of the infection, may likewise have early menopause. This situation is handed over in families.

You can examine hereditary testing choices with your primary care physician assuming you have untimely menopause or on the other hand if you have relatives who had untimely menopause.

Immune system sicknesses

Untimely menopause can be a side effect of an immune system illness, like thyroid sickness or rheumatoid joint inflammation.

In immune system sicknesses, the safe framework confuses a piece of the body with a trespasser and assaults it. Irritation brought about by a portion of these infections can influence the ovaries. Menopause starts when the ovaries quit working.

Epilepsy
Epilepsy is a seizure problem that stems from the mind. Somebody with epilepsy is bound to encounter essential ovarian deficiency, which prompts menopause. Changing chemical levels because of menopause can influence seizures in individuals with epilepsy.

A more established study from 2001 tracked down that in a gathering of ladies with epilepsy, around 14% of those contemplated had untimely menopause, rather than 1% of everyone.

Could early menopause at any point add to different circumstances?
Fruitlessness is much of the time a major concern when you start menopause at least 10 years ahead of schedule. However, there are other wellbeing concerns.

A constant flow of estrogen to your tissues has many purposes. Estrogen increments "great" HDL cholesterol and diminishes "terrible" LDL cholesterol. It additionally loosens up veins and keeps bones from diminishing.

Losing estrogen sooner than run-of-the-mill can expand your gamble of:

coronary illness
osteoporosis
sadness
dementia
sudden passing
Assuming that you have worries about these side effects, talk with your PCP. On account of these dangers, individuals who enter menopause early are often recommended HRT.

Could early menopause at any point safeguard you from different circumstances?
Beginning menopause early can shield you from different infections. These incorporate estrogen-delicate malignant growths like a bosom disease.

Individuals who enter menopause late (after age 55) are at a more serious gamble of bosom malignant growth than the people who enter the change prior. This is because their bosom tissue is presented to estrogen for a more drawn-out time frame.
Facilitating the progress to menopause
A hereditary test may one day decide an individual's probability of early menopause. For the present,

however, the truth will come out eventually when you begin your change.

Contact your PCP for customary exams, and attempt to be proactive about your conceptive well-being. Doing so can assist your primary care physician with facilitating the side effects or abatement of your gamble factors for early menopause.

Seeing a specialist can likewise assist you with adapting to any aggravation or nervousness you might feel during menopause.

Richness and your choices
If you're keen on having kids, you have a couple of choices for developing your loved ones. These include:

reception
getting an egg gift
having a substitute convey your kid
A fruitfulness expert may likewise recommend strategies that can assist you with having kids. Consult with your PCP about the choices accessible to you for becoming a parent. Their dangers and victories can be impacted by many elements, including your age and by and large well-being.

HOW IS EARLY MENOPAUSE ANALYZED?

The time driving into menopause is called perimenopause. During this time, you might have sporadic periods and different side effects that go back and forth.

You're for the most part viewed as in menopause if you go a year without feminine dying, and you don't have one more ailment to make sense of your side effects. This might be a sign of early menopause.

Testing for early menopause
Tests aren't generally expected to analyze menopause. A great many people can self-analyze menopause given their side effects. In any case, if you believe you're encountering early menopause, you might need to contact your PCP no doubt.

Your PCP can arrange chemical tests to assist with deciding if your side effects are expected to perimenopause or another condition. These are the most well-known chemicals to check:

Against Müllerian chemical (AMH). The PicoAMH Elisa test utilizes this chemical to assist with deciding if you're moving toward menopause or have previously arrived at your last period.

Estrogen. Your primary care physician might take a look at your degrees of estrogen, likewise called estradiol. In menopause, estrogen levels decline.
Follicle-invigorating chemical (FSH). Assuming your FSH levels are reliably over 30 milli-global units per milliliter (mIU/mL), and you haven't been discharged for a year, all things considered, you've arrived at menopause. Nonetheless, a solitary raised FSH test can't affirm menopause all alone.
Thyroid-animating chemical (TSH). Your primary care physician might really look at your degrees of TSH to affirm analysis. Assuming you have an underactive thyroid (hypothyroidism), you'll have TSH levels that are excessively high. Side effects of the condition are like the side effects of menopause.
The North American Menopause Society (NAMS) reports that chemical tests are now and again pointless because chemical levels change and vacillate during perimenopause.

All things considered, if you're worried about indications of menopause, NAMS recommends mentioning a full exam with your primary care physician.
How is early menopause treated or made due?
Early menopause by and large doesn't need treatment.

Notwithstanding, there are treatment choices accessible to assist with dealing with the side effects of menopause or conditions connected with it. They can assist you with managing changes in your body or way of life all the more without any problem.

Untimely menopause is frequently treated because it happens at such an early age. This assists support your body with the chemicals it would ordinarily make until you arrive at the period of regular menopause.

The most widely recognized treatment incorporates chemical substitution treatment (HRT). Foundational chemical treatment can forestall numerous normal menopausal side effects. Or on the other hand, you might take vaginal chemical items, typically in low portions, to assist with vaginal side effects.

However, HRT has gambles. It can build your possibilities of:

coronary illness
stroke
bosom disease
Consult with your PCP about the dangers and advantages of your singular consideration prior to beginning HRT. Lower portions of chemicals might diminish your gamble of encountering these circumstances.

Way of life and home cures
Even though you can't keep menopause from occurring, you can make a move to help your side effects.

Eating a solid eating routine and practicing consistently can assist with overseeing menopause side effects. On the off chance that you smoke, consider stopping to deal with your side effects.

There is blended proof of utilizing normal items to oversee menopause side effects. Certain individuals lean toward nutrients and homegrown supplements over regular medicine. Check with your PCP about which treatment is ideal for you.

Could early menopause at any point be turned around? For the time being, accessible treatment can help delay or diminish the side effects of menopause, however, there is no certain method for turning around early menopause.

In any case, specialists are exploring better approaches to assist people in menopause who have youngsters.

In 2016, researchers in Greece declared another treatment that empowered them to reestablish periods and recover eggs from a little gathering of ladies who were in perimenopause.

This treatment stood out as truly newsworthy as a way to "switch" menopause, yet little is realized about how well it functions.

The researchers revealed treating more than 30 ladies, ages 46 to 49, by infusing platelet-rich plasma (PRP) into their ovaries. PRP is some of the time used to advance tissue mending, yet the treatment isn't successful for any reason.

The researchers guaranteed the treatment worked for 66% of the ladies treated. Notwithstanding, the examination has been condemned for its small size and absence of control gatherings.

However the examination could have potential for the future, it's anything but a sensible treatment choice at this moment.

How is early menopause treated or made due?
Early menopause by and large doesn't need treatment.

In any case, there are treatment choices accessible to assist with dealing with the side effects of menopause or conditions connected with it. They can assist you with managing changes in your body or way of life all the more without any problem.

Untimely menopause is frequently treated because it happens at such an early age. This assists support your body with the chemicals it would regularly make until you arrive at the period of normal menopause.

The most well-known treatment incorporates chemical substitution treatment (HRT). Fundamental chemical treatment can forestall numerous normal menopausal side effects. Or on the other hand, you might take

vaginal chemical items, for the most part in low portions, to assist with vaginal side effects.
Notwithstanding, analysts are exploring better approaches to assist people in menopause who have youngsters.

In 2016, researchers in Greece declared another treatment that empowered them to reestablish the feminine cycle and recover eggs from a little gathering of ladies who were in perimenopause.
This treatment stood out as truly newsworthy as a way to "switch" menopause, yet little is realized about how well it functions.

The researchers announced treating over 30 ladies, ages 46 to 49, by infusing platelet-rich plasma (PRP) into their ovaries. PRP is at times used to advance tissue mending, however, the treatment isn't compelling for any reason.

The researchers guaranteed the treatment worked for 66% of the ladies treated. Notwithstanding, the exploration has been scrutinized for its small size and absence of control gatherings.

However the examination could have potential for the future, it's anything but a practical treatment choice at present.

SEMI-SUMMARY

Menopause is characterized as the super-durable end of menses coming about because of decreased ovarian chemical emission that happens normally or is prompted by a medical procedure, chemotherapy, or radiation. Regular menopause is perceived following a year of amenorrhea that isn't related to a pathologic reason. The typical period of menopause in the US is 51 years and can change ordinarily somewhere in the range of 40 and 58 years.1 The menopausal progress can traverse north for quite a while, and frequently starts with varieties in monthly cycle length in light of rising degrees of follicle animating chemical (FSH). The mean time of the beginning of the menopausal progress is 47.5 years and normally endures roughly 4 to 5 years.

Stages and classification of the menopausal change were characterized by specialists in 2001 at the Phases of Regenerative Maturing Studio (STRAW).2 The gathering perceived seven phases of the conceptive maturing continuum and recognized that most ladies don't advance definitively through each stage. These stages are additionally portrayed by the accompanying terms:

Premenopause: the time up to the start of the perimenopause, but on the other hand is utilized to characterize the time up to the last feminine period.
Perimenopause: the time around menopause during which feminine cycle and endocrine changes are happening yet a year of amenorrhea has not yet happened.
Postmenopause: starts at the
 hour of the last feminine time frame, albeit not perceived until following a year of amenorrhea.

A hot glimmer or flush alludes to the unconstrained impression of warmth, frequently connected with sweat, coming about because of a vasomotor reaction to declining estrogen levels. Night sweats are hot glimmers or flushes happening around evening time, frequently while resting. Different side effects, like vaginal dryness, rest aggravation, mindset side effects, mental unsettling influences, substantial grumblings, urinary objections, uterine draining issues, sexual brokenness, and decreased personal satisfaction are additionally credited to the menopausal progress.

Although many measures have been created to survey menopausal side effects, few exhibit normalization, legitimacy, or unwavering quality. A few measures depend on self-reports of the presence, seriousness, and recurrence of individual side effects, like hot glimmers. Others use aggregate or worldwide scores given records or sizes of side effects credited to menopause, like state of mind, perception, personal satisfaction, sexual capability, and physical side effects. Many investigations base their actions on study-specific agendas, polls, or scales. Ninety-two proportions of menopausal side effects were accounted for by concentrates on remembered for this proof survey.

Reason
This deliberate proof survey centers around five Key Inquiries connecting with the side effects of menopause and their administration, as determined by the Arranging Council for the Public Organizations of Wellbeing State-of-the-Science Meeting on Administration of Menopause-Related Side Effects. The objective populace remembers grown-up individuals from the US going through the menopausal process.

What is the proof that the side effects all the more often detailed by middle-aged ladies are inferable from ovarian maturing and senescence?
These include:
Vasomotor side effects.
Vaginal dryness.
Rest unsettling influence.
Mindset side effects.
Mental unsettling influences.
Substantial objections.
Urinary grievances.
Uterine draining issues.
Sexual brokenness.
Diminished personal satisfaction.

When do the menopausal side effects show up, how long do they persevere with what recurrence and seriousness, and why are the elements that impact they known?
Factors include:
Race and identity.
Age at beginning of the menopause progress.
Weight record (BMI).
Careful versus regular menopause.
Melancholy.
Smoking.
What is the proof for the advantages and damages of normally involved intercessions for alleviation of menopause-related side effects?
Mediations include:
Estrogens.
Progestins.
Androgens.
Tibolone.
Antidepressants.
Different medications.
Phytoestrogens.
Corresponding and elective medication.
Social intercessions.
What are the significant contemplations in overseeing menopause-related side effects in ladies with clinical attributes or conditions that might entangle decision-making?
These include:
Two-sided oophorectomy.
Untimely ovarian disappointment.

Bosom malignant growth.
Simultaneous utilization of particular estrogen receptor modulators (SERMs) and other interfacing restorative specialists.
Way of life and conduct factors.
Late stopping of menopausal chemical treatment.
Exceptionally low or extremely high BMI.
What are the future exploration headings for treatment of menopause-related side effects and conditions?
Techniques
A Specialized Master Board was collected to give input from specialists and clinicians in the field to guarantee that the extent of the task resolved significant clinical inquiries and issues. The board included obstetricians/gynecologists, internists, naturopathic doctors, social specialists, and analysts. The board was assembled for occasional phone calls throughout the venture. Master analysts, including a few board individuals, gave remarks on the draft proof report.

Writing Search and Procedure
Important investigations were recognized from numerous hunts of MEDLINE®, PsycINFO, DARE, the Cochrane data set of methodical surveys and controlled preliminaries, MANTIS, and AMED (1953 to November 2004); and from late deliberate audits, reference records, surveys, articles, sites, and specialists. Recovered abstracts were placed into an electronic data set (EndNote®).

Incorporation and Avoidance Rules

Full message companion studies with information on ladies encountering menopause and somewhere around one of the side effects recorded in Key Inquiry 1 were at first audited and hence included assuming the review enlisted at least 100 subjects, subjects addressed the objective populace, and information on side effects related with menopause was given. Prohibitions included investigations of ladies not going through the menopausal change and encountering menopause-related side effects, investigations of maturing and its belongings, and organically based examinations that didn't report epidemiological information connecting with side effects (e.g., investigations of chemical levels). Non-English language papers and investigations of creatures or dead bodies were additionally rejected. Cross-sectional concentrates on gathering comparable consideration/rejection measures were inspected for contributory information and included if they detailed important information about side effects by menopausal stage, for example, predominance rates.

Full-text randomized controlled preliminaries and meta-analyses of randomized controlled preliminaries giving information on the treatment of menopausal side effects, utilizing at least one of the mediations recorded in Key Inquiry 3, were incorporated. Preliminaries selecting ladies with bosom malignant growth were thought about independently from those enlisting ladies without bosom disease. Prohibitions included investigations of ladies not going through menopause and encountering menopause-related side effects over the span of the review, investigations of creatures, and non-English language papers.

Information Extraction and Blend
All qualified examinations were surveyed and a "best proof" approach was applied, in which studies with the greatest and most thorough plan are emphasized.3 Information was extricated from each review, entered straightforwardly into proof tables, and summed up distinctly. Benefits and unfriendly impacts of treatments were viewed as similarly significant and the two sorts of results were preoccupied. Preliminaries of option and integral treatments were assembled by the Public Community for Correlative and Elective Medication categories4 most firmly connected with included subjects. Aftereffects of as of late-distributed meta-analyses on estrogens5-7 and isoflavones8 are remembered for this report. No new meta-analyses were led due to the heterogeneity of preliminaries of different treatments.

Two analysts autonomously evaluated the nature of randomized controlled preliminaries and companion concentrates on utilizing measures well defined for various review plans created by the US Preventive Administrations Undertaking Force.9 Comparable standards for cross-sectional studies are not accessible. The general rating is a mix of inner and outer legitimacy scores. At the point when commentators dissented, a last evaluation was arrived at through agreement. Concentrates on detailing a few unique results might have different quality evaluations for every result contingent upon how it controlled for key confounders in multivariable models.

Size of Writing
A sum of 10,059 one-of-a-kind references were checked on, including 6,342 about side effects and factors impacting them (Key Inquiries 1 and 2); 4,078 about treatments (Key Inquiry 3); and 806 about unambiguous qualities that might impact the impacts of treatments (Key Inquiry 4).

Results
To resolve Key Inquiries 1 and 2, the audit zeroed in on planned investigations of associates of midlife ladies progressing through the phases of menopause. Forty-eight investigations directed among 14 partners met consideration measures. Seven accomplices were situated in the US (Massachusetts Ladies' Wellbeing Study, Seattle Midlife Ladies' Wellbeing Study, Ohio Midlife Ladies' Review, Public Wellbeing Assessment Follow-up Study [NHANES], Investigation of Ladies' Wellbeing The country over [SWAN], College of Minnesota/Tremin Trust Longitudinal Review, and Pennsylvania Ovarian Maturing Study). Seven associates were based external the US (Gothenburg, Sweden, Australian Longitudinal Concentrate on Ladies' Wellbeing, Clinical Exploration Chamber [MRC], U.K., Melbourne Ladies' Midlife Wellbeing Undertaking, Australia, Manitoba Venture on Ladies and Their Wellbeing in the Center Years, Canada, Copenhagen,

Denmark, and Eindhoven, Netherlands). 22 extra cross-sectional studies from different populations meeting comparative consideration standards were acquired to give extra pervasiveness information.

Significant impediments of studies incorporate different strategies for assessing and detailing side effects and for surveying menopausal change. Some partner concentrates on putting together outcomes concerning cross-sectional information revealed at a sequential time focus as opposed to individual following of ladies after some time. A few examinations neglected to change or separate for possibly significant factors like age, race, BMI, life-altering situations, or history of gloom while endeavoring to credit side effects to change in the menopausal stage.

Albeit most included examinations were population-based, much of the time, enlisted ladies were furthermore chosen from the underlying enrolled accomplice and may have been less delegate of everybody. Likewise, many examinations depended on companions enrolled from local area populaces and are more agents of workers than whole networks.

Key Inquiry 1. What is the proof that the side effects all the more often detailed by middle-aged ladies are inferable from ovarian maturing and senescence? Vasomotor side effects: Proof from a population-based accomplice and cross-sectional concentrates on upholding the relationship between vasomotor side effects and the menopausal stage. Studies are predictable in detailing expanding pervasiveness paces of vasomotor side effects as ladies change from premenopause to either perimenopause or postmenopause, influencing 50% or a greater amount of ladies. Studies propose that vasomotor side effects persevere for a long time after menopause for certain ladies.

Vaginal dryness: Vaginal dryness is related to menopause and pervasiveness rates increment as ladies progress through the menopausal stages. Gauges show that dependent upon
 33% of perimenopausal and postmenopausal ladies experience vaginal dryness.

Rest unsettling influence: Even though the consequences of studies are blended, two good-quality companion studies show that ladies have more trouble dozing as they change through menopausal stages, and this might be because of vasomotor side effects. Up to 40 percent to 60 percent of perimenopausal and postmenopausal ladies experience rest unsettling influence, a slight increment from the pervasiveness paces of premenopausal ladies.

State of mind side effects: most studies from an enormous writing report no relationship between menopausal stage and temperament side effects, improvement of a psychological problem, or general emotional well-being. Investigations of commonness rates report wide ranges that are comparable across menopausal stages.

Mental unsettling influences: No associate investigations are accessible. Cross-sectional studies show no distinction in neglect, memory, or fixation.

Substantial grumblings: Most examinations report no relationship between physical side effects with menopause, albeit physical side effects were expanded among perimenopausal ladies contrasted and premenopausal ladies in a single partner and two cross-sectional studies.

Urinary objections: Urinary spillage expanded among perimenopausal ladies contrasted and premenopausal ladies in a single report and one more detailed no affiliations. Investigations of predominance rates report wide ranges that are comparative across menopausal stages.

Uterine draining issues: No examinations meeting consideration rules tended to uterine draining issues, doubtlessly because presently acknowledged meanings of menopause depend generally on changes in uterine dying.

Sexual brokenness: Ladies from one review partner detailed decreases in some or each of the deliberate sexual boundaries as they progressed through the menopausal stages. The consequences of cross-sectional studies are blended.

Diminished personal satisfaction: Aftereffects of accessible partner and cross-sectional studies are clashing.

Key Inquiry 2. When do the menopausal side effects show up, how long do they continue with what recurrence and seriousness, and why are the elements that impact they known?

Included investigations don't give satisfactory subtleties to describe the beginning, seriousness, and term of explicit side effects. Recurrence is depicted by pervasiveness information in Key Inquiry 1.

Race and nationality: The impact of race and identity on menopausal side effects has not been broadly examined. Predominance paces of vasomotor and temperament side effects shift among race and ethnic gatherings in the huge SWAN companion.

Age at the beginning of menopausal change: Accessible investigations are uncertain.

Weight file: Accessible examinations are uncertain.

Careful versus regular menopause: Studies present blended results regarding the effect of careful menopause on vasomotor side effects, vaginal dryness, and temperament. Change for confounders is fundamental since ladies going through hysterectomy contrast from ladies with normal menopause in manners that may likewise impact their menopause-related side effects.

Discouragement: One cross-sectional review revealed that earlier uneasiness or sorrow didn't foresee menopausal side effects. Partner concentrates on showing that a past filled with gloom predicts sadness in the menopausal progress. No examinations assessed discouragement in association with other menopausal side effects.

Smoking: Accessible investigations are uncertain.

Key Inquiry 3. What is the proof for the advantages and damages of generally involved intercessions for the help of menopause-related side effects?

A sum of 192 randomized controlled preliminaries of treatments for overseeing menopause-related side effects was assessed, including preliminaries of estrogens, progestins, androgens (testosterone and DHEA [dehydroepiandrosterone]), tibolone, antidepressants (particularly serotonin reuptake inhibitors, moclobemide, veralipride), different medications (clonidine, methyldopa, gabapentin, Bellergal), phytoestrogens (dietary and concentrate types of soy isoflavones, different types of phytoestrogen, blends), corresponding and elective medication (needle therapy, Chinese spices, red clover, dark cohosh, mixes, different sorts of enhancements, manual treatments, energy treatments), and conduct intercessions (practice and different kinds of mediations).

Estrogen, in either going against or unopposed regimens, is the most reliably compelling treatment for vasomotor side effects and shows benefit in many preliminaries assessing urogenital side effects. Some, however not all, preliminaries assessing rest, temperament and sorrow, sexual capability, and personal satisfaction results likewise report benefits with estrogen contrasted with fake treatment.

Bosom delicacy and uterine draining are the most ordinarily announced unfavorable results in estrogen preliminaries; others incorporate sickness and regurgitating, migraine, weight change, wooziness, venous thromboembolic occasions, cardiovascular occasions, rash and pruritus, cholecystitis, and liver impacts.

Preliminaries of progestin demonstrate blended results for the treatment of vasomotor side effects.

Not many preliminaries of testosterone are accessible; one preliminary demonstrated no distinctions between testosterone/estrogen and estrogen alone for hot blaze seriousness, vaginal dryness, or rest issues. Sexual side effects were improved with testosterone/estrogen contrasted with estrogen alone or fake treatment in two different preliminaries.

For ladies utilizing testosterone joined with estrogen, skin breaks out and hirsutism happens essentially more frequently than for ladies utilizing estrogen alone.

In light of a couple of fair or good-quality preliminaries, tibolone showed benefit for vasomotor side effects, rest, and physical grievances contrasted with fake treatment, and was like estrogen for some, however not all, side effects.

Uterine dying, body torment, weight gain, and migraine were more normal in tibolone versus fake treatment gatherings.

A few specialists exhibit benefits in overseeing vasomotor side effects in some, yet not all preliminaries, or in a couple of accessible preliminaries, including paroxetine, veralipride, gabapentin, soy isoflavones, and other phytoestrogens.

Preliminaries of soy isoflavones and other correlative and elective medication treatments report benefits in improving nonvasomotor side effects, even though results change broadly, strategies are missing, and studies are normally little and not generalizable. Self-influenced consequences in preliminaries are huge reflecting basic vacillations of side effects.

Even though the advantages and unfriendly impacts of treatments were similarly significant in this audit, most preliminaries didn't report antagonistic impacts or detail them completely.

Key Inquiry 4. What are the significant contemplations in overseeing menopause-related side effects in ladies with clinical qualities or conditions that might confound decision-making?

The proof isn't accessible to decide whether the adequacy of treatment for menopause-related side effects or unfriendly impacts contrast for ladies with reciprocal oophorectomy, untimely ovarian disappointment, simultaneous utilization of SERMs or other possibly cooperating specialists, way of life and conduct factors, ongoing end of menopausal chemical treatment, or exceptionally low or extremely high BMI. For ladies with bosom disease, consequences of 15 randomized controlled preliminaries show that clonidine, venlafaxine, and megestrol acetic acid derivation are related with fundamentally further developed proportions of hot glimmers, and vitamin E, dark cohosh, isoflavones, magnets, and fluoxetine are not. Results for nonvasomotor results are blended.

Key Inquiry 5. What are the future exploration headings for treatment of menopause-related side effects and conditions?

To fill proof holes, future exploration could zero in on:

Assurance of ideally successful dosages, mix regimens, spans of purpose, and timing of treatment.
Assessment of ways to deal with recognizes ideal contenders for explicit treatments (e.g., ID of thrombophilias).
Head-to-head and fake treatment examinations of estrogen alone and joined with different sorts of treatments including non-drug intercessions.
Preliminaries exhibit how to cease estrogen when side effects die down, including the viability of tightening dosages as well as supplanting with different treatments including non-drug mediations.
Better announcing antagonistic impacts in preliminaries and utilization of normalized classes of unfavorable impacts so information can be consolidated across preliminaries.
Further developed examination of results including investigation by hysterectomy and oophorectomy status, phase of menopause, age, simultaneous circumstances and prescriptions, and different variables.
More exhaustive preliminaries to decide the job of normal activity, rest the executives, ideal sustenance, solid connections, social help, and unwinding; impacts of mind-body methods like biofeedback and breathing; impacts of an entire framework approach with Chinese medication.
Extra, well-designed, and controlled preliminaries of phytoestrogens, botanicals, and bio-identical chemicals, particularly estriol, estradiol, and progesterone. Further

investigation of antidepressants for vasomotor side effects would be legitimate in light of proof of right now accessible preliminaries.

Enlistment of ladies with explicit attributes who have not recently been assessed, for example, nonwhite ladies, ladies with untimely ovarian disappointment, those utilizing SERMs and different specialists impacting side effects simultaneously, ladies with extremely high or low BMI, and those with way of life and conduct factors affecting side effects. Preliminaries ought to report information well-defined for these gatherings to decipher their effect on treatment.

Utilization of standard definitions, measures, results, and factual techniques for longitudinal information so results can be measured across preliminaries and populace accomplices.

Predominance information in U.S. ladies.

Insights concerning the beginning, timing, and span of side effects comparable to the menopausal stage.

Investigations of side effects after careful menopause with and without hormonal treatment.

SUMMARY

In view of a survey of presently accessible companion and crossectional populace studies, vasomotor side effects and vaginal dryness are side effects generally reliably connected with menopausal change. Rest aggravation, physical objections, urinary grumblings, sexual brokenness, temperament, and personal satisfaction are conflictingly related. No accomplice studies give information on perception, yet cross-sectional studies recommend no affiliation. There are no examinations about uterine draining issues, beginning, span, and seriousness of explicit side effects, or indisputable information because of race/identity, period of beginning of menopause, BMI, oophorectomy status, presence of wretchedness, or smoking status. The writing is restricted by contrasts in how side effects are characterized and estimated, changeability of study populaces, and contradiction of information forestalling direct correlations between studies or pooling of results. Future examination involving standard and approved measures and uniform definitions for a more far-reaching exhibit of side effects would further develop information on these affiliations.

Preliminaries of treatment are decisive just for estrogen and its utilization in treating vasomotor and urogenital side effects, albeit different treatments might demonstrate powerful if further examined. Undertaking preliminaries to treat side effects that are not connected with the menopausal change wouldn't be helpful. Preliminaries are restricted in numerous ways including:

Utilization of profoundly chosen little examples of ladies. Brief terms.
Deficient detailing of misfortune to follow up, support of similar gatherings, tainting, strategies for examination, and unfavorable occasions.
Utilization of divergent measures and results that are frequently not normalized or approved.
Indistinct incorporation and rejection measures.
Industry sponsorship.
Future examination tending to these lacks, as framed in Key Inquiry 5, would direct quiet and clinician decision-making while overseeing menopause-related side effects.

The proof survey is restricted in more ways than one. For Key Inquiries 1 and 2, writing look-through zeroed in on populace investigations of ladies going through the menopausal change announcing side effects and did exclude epidemiologic or biologically-based etiologic examinations. Likewise, concentrates on those that might not have been distinguished via look remember those for which menopause was not an essential focal point of the review, but rather an indicator variable remembered for a multivariable model assessing the result or side effect of interest. Concentrates on possibly not distinguished would be those that recognized no relationship between the menopausal stage and the result of interest. Studies with a positive affiliation would likely have detailed it in the theoretical and be distinguished by the pursuits. Additionally, the audit was restricted to English language randomized controlled preliminaries of treatments.